acts
of
friend-
ship

47 WAYS
TO RECHARGE YOUR LIFE,
MAKE *REAL* CONNECTIONS,
AND DEEPEN YOUR
RELATIONSHIPS

acts of friend- ship

LYNNE EVERATT,
DEB MANGOLT, AND
JULIE SMETHURST

● PAGE
● TWO
BOOKS

Cataloguing in publication information is available from Library and Archives Canada.

ISBN 978-1-989025-97-0 (paperback)
ISBN 978-1-989025-98-7 (ebook)

Page Two
www.pagetwo.com

Cover design by Peter Cocking
Author photo by Marta Hewson
Cover illustration by Michelle Clement
Interior design by Setareh Ashrafologhalai
Printed and bound in Canada by Friesens
Distributed in Canada by Raincoast Books
Distributed in the US and internationally by Publishers Group West, a division of Ingram

20 21 22 23 24   5 4 3 2 1

actsoffriendship.com

This book is not intended as a substitute for the medical advice of physicians. The reader should regularly consult a physician in matters relating to his/her health and particularly with respect to any symptoms that may require diagnosis or medical attention.

*To women who raise each other
up through friendship*

Contents

II. Acts of Creativity

III. Acts of Adventure

Before the First Act

"Good relationships keep us
happier and healthier. Period."
ROBERT WALDINGER

HAVE YOU EVER considered the importance of the friendships in your life, and that nurturing those relationships could be one of the *best* things you can do for your mental *and* physical health? The Harvard Study of Adult Development has been tracking people since 1938—the longest-running study on life and happiness in the world—and has uncovered this surprising finding that we wish was common knowledge: people who were the most satisfied in their relationships at age fifty were the healthiest at age eighty. Friendships are a better predictor of health than cholesterol levels. And not only do good relationships protect our bodies, but they also protect our brains. People with strong social ties are proven to experience less mental decline as they age. More than money, fame, or the total number of social media "likes," close relationships keep people happy throughout their lives. "The key to healthy aging," according to Harvard researcher George Vaillant, "is relationships, relationships, relationships."

For far too many people, the world has become a sad, angry, and anxious place. Is it any coincidence that we are also increasingly lonely? Research shows that socially isolated people have a significantly increased risk of premature death compared to those who have stronger interpersonal bonds. Being disconnected reverberates through our minds and bodies, and has been compared to the health-destroying effects of smoking fifteen cigarettes a day. Loneliness kills.

We know that relationships are good for us, but maintaining (or deepening) our friendships often falls to the bottom of our priority lists as we chase other measures of success that appear to have more attractive, résumé-boosting payoffs. In their book *The Lonely American*, Harvard psychiatry professors Jacqueline Olds and Richard Schwartz describe the rise of loneliness and a decline in meaningful relationships: the push of "productivity and the cult of busyness" along with a desire to stage-manage our relationships through the filtering lens of social media are pulling us apart. Real relationships take time, care, and physical presence: there are no social media shortcuts, no hacks, no other ways to build relationships than to repeatedly make the choice to show up and pay attention. Wearable technologies can't compare to real-life friends when it comes to helping us make positive behavioral changes. A hiking boot badge for hitting 25,000 steps in a day will never give us the same boost as a hug from a friend at the end of the trail, yet many people continue to ignore the benefits of real, in-person community.

To determine how many *real* relationships people have, the General Social Survey, a group headed by Duke University researcher Miller McPherson, asked people face-to-face, "Looking back over the last six months, who are the people with whom you discussed matters important to you?" followed up with the lie detector: "What are their first names or initials?" The survey found that between 1985 and 2004, the number of people with whom Americans discussed important matters dropped from three to two, and more startlingly, the number of people who said they had *no* confidants tripled, making up nearly a quarter of respondents.

We may think that with hundreds of social media connections we can't possibly be lonely, but when it comes to relationships that comfort and uplift us, social media doesn't cut it. Sherry Turkle, an MIT professor and a clinical psychologist, is deeply concerned about how social media is affecting interpersonal closeness. Turkle isn't anti-technology, she's pro-conversation, and she worries that a generation that chooses text over talk has lost the ability to listen, learn about, and understand each other. And, Turkle asserts, when we miss out on conversations with others while using technology to avoid ever being alone with our thoughts, we lose the ability to relate to *ourselves*. Hundreds of Facebook friends aren't as valuable as true friends—people with whom you can have face-to-face conversations and feel comfortable being yourself, or people with whom you feel safe enough to try your hand at being someone completely different. It's not the number of friends you have, but the *quality* of your close relationships that matters.

Acts of Friendship offers a remedy for disconnection. It's an entire book about how you can intentionally deepen your close relationships to transform your life for the better. Each chapter describes an enjoyable activity that friends can do together, backed by research supporting its health benefits. You might want to approach the book as a spin on a book club, taking turns designing monthly or weekly activities from the chapter of your choice. Although our intended audience is women, we'd love it if men would engage in a few of the activities as well—especially A Woman's Rite, which will encourage them to commune with divine feminine energy.

We are three women who met and became friends when we worked together for the same multinational company. As our friendships grew, so did our desire to get more out of life: we wanted our lives to be more closely aligned with the things we loved. All the self-help books tell you to find your passion and follow your bliss, but often your talents come so naturally to you that they don't feel like talents at all. You need a friend to tell you that you're exceptional and that your talent is worth pursuing on a grander scale. And you need more than one approach to expand your concept of who you are and what's possible—this is where our acts of friendship have helped us and can help you, too.

We have tested more than one hundred activities on our own friend dates, including Horsing Around in which Deb was thrown off Joey the runaway stallion (we excluded that one!) and Pop Art in which we attempted to create random masterpieces by smashing balloons filled with paint that were pinned to a canvas (we excluded that one as well!) to select the forty-seven most enjoyable, beneficial, and accessible activities for *Acts of Friendship*. The acts are designed to broaden your perspective, expose your true self, build courage, and change your life in ways you never expected. It's no coincidence that our lives expanded in tandem with our get-togethers. By engaging in purposeful activities in an intentional way, we discovered a formula for personal growth that produced moments of meaning where our random yearnings and aimless wanderings finally made sense. And we all know that when you hit upon those "aha" moments—like when you discover that you'd rather be a pastry chef than an investment banker—you have to share them with your friends.

Our experience of friendship as a catalyst for life change isn't unique. People have always looked to one another for encouragement and guidance, and today the need to connect and make sense of it all is greater than ever. Whenever and wherever people gather with their friends—even if it's just around the corner for an evening without partners or children—they are responding to an urge to converge that is backed up by an ever-growing accumulation of research: friendships help fight illness and depression, speed recovery, slow aging, and prolong life.

When we initially planned our get-togethers we weren't aware of the research data on friendships. All we knew was that whenever we met, our lives improved. As active women caught up in careers and family obligations, we had a desire to get more out of life, and more out of our limited time together. We wanted to experience lots of rejuvenating laughter, to create more opportunities to encourage each other, to expand our horizons... and to give back. So rather than simply getting together for a tidy block of catch-up time, which sometimes felt like a "wine-y" work meeting, we decided to take our get-togethers one step further. We looked at the latest research on what makes a happy and fulfilling life, and designed our activities to maximize the benefits of getting together.

Personal growth disguised as a friendly get-together—is it possible?

We discovered the answer to this question is an emphatic *yes*. Self-improvement is best enjoyed with friends who can help each other acknowledge potential and reach those places of greatness within ourselves that we know are there, but were previously inaccessible. Friends offer the gentle reassurance that we don't have to let the past determine the future, and that it's enough for us to become better than we are today, according to our own yardstick. We've helped each other understand that we don't have to *do* or *have* the most, but that we can each become our best selves and have some fun along the way.

Our friendly get-togethers became life-shifting experiences. While performing A Night at the Improv, we learned that our listening skills can be joyfully sharpened. When we tried out Thank You, Thank You, Thank You, we discovered that the proven health benefits of expressing gratitude can be multiplied when done collectively. Through our experiences in reflection, we acknowledged that the inner child found in Childhood Excavations could be a great teacher. Creative activities such as Standing Jokes and Think on Your Stilettos revealed hidden talents, and Ages Eight and Up made at least one of us realize that she should stick to her day job. Our adventures in exploring other cultures and religions revealed what shared humanity feels like. Everything we experienced by participating in the activities found in this book gave us memories that will last a lifetime and an awareness of what matters—which we might never have achieved on our own. We are thrilled to be able to share our methods and experiences with you and hope to inspire you to create your own scrapbook of memories.

The activities in *Acts of Friendship* are short projects, exercises, or excursions, most of which are free and all of which are inspiring. As you perform each act, you may find it desirable to keep a journal to record your moments of insight on your unique path to self-discovery and personal growth.

The book is divided into three sections: reflection, creativity, and adventure.

- **Reflection activities.** These encourage self-awareness to help us make sense of the past and see a brighter future in which we can be ourselves, only better. They often involve learning something new, experiencing something old and familiar in a new way, or seeing ourselves through the loving perspective of a dear friend.

- **Creative activities.** These cultivate playfulness. The focus is on letting loose and having fun. Silliness rules and we abandon self-consciousness.

- **Adventure activities.** These embolden us to do what we may hesitate to try alone, exploring new places, people, and things. Adventure challenges our bodies, invites the unexpected, and expands our concept of what's possible.

This collection of inspirational activities is intended to be a wellspring of ideas for people who want to harness the power and potency of friendship. The perfect get-together companion, *Acts of Friendship* is dedicated to encouraging new adventures, discovering fresh insights, and enjoying great times with your friends. Activities have been designed to give you the most value for the least money in the shortest amount of time.

In her book *Frientimacy*, friendship expert Shasta Nelson describes the three key elements of a healthy, vibrant relationship: consistency, vulnerability, and positivity. If you provide the consistency with regular friend dates, *Acts of Friendship* can add a heaping helping of positivity along with plenty of opportunities for you and your friends to share your thoughts and feelings with each other in an open, accepting, and gratifying way.

Our mission is to inspire and energize you to support each other, to reduce stress, to increase personal growth, and to have fun. We hope that the activities in *Acts of Friendship* deepen your relationships, enrich your life, and create lasting memories, just as they did for us.

Here's to raising each other up through friendship,
LYNNE, DEB, AND JULIE

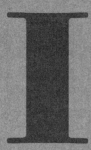

I

acts of reflection

"All that we are is the result
of what we have thought."

BUDDHA

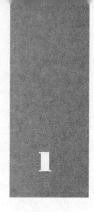

Take Your Cue

FOLLOW YOUR LOVES
TO A BETTER LIFE

"I don't believe people are looking for the meaning of life as much as they are looking for the experience of being alive."
JOSEPH CAMPBELL

HOW IMPORTANT IS it to do what you *love* rather than spending day after day doing what you're only *content* to do? Will you be happier and live longer if you do what you love? Lissa Rankin, author of *Your Inner Pilot Light*, says that the most important medicine for mind *and* body is doing what fulfills and excites you: doing what you love lights you up, she says, and turns on your natural self-healing mechanism. In her TEDx talk, Rankin explains the science behind how the state of your life affects the state of your body. Her advice is to listen to your body's "whispers" before they turn into life-threatening "screams," and to trust your inner guidance.

Take Your Cue is about turning up the volume on the small voice inside that knows what you love, allowing its guidance to take you to the place where there is joy, and then using this joy to discover the activities that fill you with a sense of purpose. According to a study published in the *Journal of the American Medical Association*, a sense of purposefulness is associated with a longer lifespan. Over the course of the five-year study, people without a purpose were significantly more likely to die during that period than people with an aim in life that they loved and that excited them. *Ikigai* (pronounced *icky-guy*) is a Japanese concept meaning "the reason for getting up in the morning." Having an *ikigai* is believed to be one of the reasons why the people of the Japanese island of Okinawa often live well into their nineties and beyond.

To begin this exciting journey of loving self-discovery that could potentially lead to a longer life, get together with your friends and a stack of blank cue cards (also known as index cards). Write "I LOVE..." at the top of each card in big, bold, capital letters and then complete the sentence with whatever comes to mind, one idea per card. Keep going without over-thinking it, writing down the things you most adore. Filling out the first few cards may feel wobbly yet strangely exhilarating and familiar, like riding a bicycle for the first time in many years. Keep at it. Eventually the inner voice that's repeating "you don't know what you love" will tire, allowing a deeper knowing to break through with new ideas. It usually takes the voice of the inner critic ten minutes or so to become hoarse, so do this activity for at least twenty minutes. Don't worry if you find it difficult: connecting with what you love, especially if you have spent many years drifting in another direction, is much harder than it looks.

After you've finished writing out your cards, take a breather. Chat with your friends about a few of your favorite things. Then, when you're feeling refreshed and ready, go back to your cue cards and organize them into piles that seem to fit together.

There are no right or wrong ways to categorize your cards, but themes in your life will begin to emerge, and you may have an "aha" moment. The benefits of Take Your Cue are twofold: first, you will be filled with gratitude for all the things you LOVE in your life; and second, you will gain perspective on the type of things you LOVE that are *missing* from your life—or that you don't have enough of.

When we did this activity together, Lynne had two business degrees and a job forecasting pharmaceuticals, but none of her cue cards professed a love of numbers or a passion for the art of exponential smoothing. Her cards did, however, spell out a deep LOVE of the arts, women's causes, and minimalist design. The activity prompted her to pursue a part-time English degree, study creative writing and acting, volunteer at a women's shelter, and throw out a whole bunch of stuff. And those cards unanimously cued her that she must somehow quit her numerical day job.

After Deb sorted her cards into themed piles, writing an objective for each stack seemed to be the next logical step. Many cards related to how much she LOVES the outdoors, and many others reflected her LOVE for physical fitness and exercise. Deb decided that one of her objectives would be to run a marathon, a goal she eventually accomplished. A simple stack of cards became the springboard to improve her health and wellbeing.

The most difficult part of this activity for Julie was waiting for the thoughts and feelings about what she LOVES to start to flow. She knew spending time with family and friends, health, learning, and adding value through work were important. But by taking time to reflect on her LOVES, a deeper truth became clear—her life was out of balance. Although she loved all the elements of her life, she saw an overemphasis on work at the expense of quality family time and self-discovery. This revelation led to a mission: she would focus less on her career, spend more time with her children, and devote more energy to personal growth. The long-term result was that she carved out a new career through part-time arrangements and a more balanced, happier life. Oh, and Julie's love of freedom propelled her to take up flying!

Whether or not you change your career or your entire lifestyle, doing more of what fulfills and excites you will improve your overall health. What will you discover about yourself and what actions will you take to bring more of the things that thrill you in your life when you Take Your Cue?

The Chuck-It List

KICK THE BUCKET LIST AND LIVE A LIFE TRUE TO YOURSELF

"Saying no can be the ultimate self-care."
CLAUDIA BLACK

MANY PEOPLE CHOOSE to create a bucket list of all the things they think they should do before they "kick the bucket." The origin of the saying "to kick the bucket" isn't clear, but it may have come from back in the day when people who were sentenced to death by hanging stood on a bucket before it was kicked out from under them. Having anything kicked out from under you isn't a pleasant experience, and a poorly designed bucket list can leave you hanging in a purgatory of unfulfilled desires. Bucket lists designed out of obligation can make you less spontaneous, lead to unrealistic expectations, and encourage you to do things that might look good in the eyes of others rather than for pleasure. That's why we propose The Chuck-It List, a list of things you *refuse* to do.

On their deathbed, few have bucket-list thoughts like, "If only I had climbed Mount Everest!" In her book *The Top Five*

Regrets of the Dying, author and former palliative care worker Bronnie Ware shares the number one regret of the dying as, "I wish I'd had the courage to live a life true to myself, not the life others expected of me." Deadly regrets don't come from missing out on once-in-a-lifetime experiences, but from repeatedly letting other people make our life choices for us. Your life consists of roughly 30,000 days and you've probably lived at least a third of them. Do you want to spend another minute doing things you and others think you *should* do? And do you want to sign up for any experience solely out of a fear of missing out?

The purpose of a chuck-it list is to eliminate constant "shoulding"—to stop thinking about what you should do but don't want to do. You can recognize shoulding behavior by the uneasy feeling it usually leaves in the pit of your stomach. The chuck-it list will cleanse you of toxic "shoulds" and the anxiety that comes along with them. Think of it as a life detox that may involve chucking an item off your bucket list along with cleansing yourself of repeated shoulding.

For example, let's say you think you should climb Mount Everest because it would be cool to tell everyone that you've done it. But first you have to fly to Kathmandu, Nepal, and from there to Lukla Airport, which is high in the Himalayas, and then walk to Namche Bazar and acclimatize to the altitude. And from there it would still take ten days just to trek to the base camp, and there's always the possibility of high-altitude cerebral edema, sudden storms, and subfreezing temperatures. Not to mention you'd have to pay the Nepalese government thousands of dollars for a permit, along with payouts to a team of guides and a cook, for a total cost that can approach a mountainous $100,000, all for the privilege of a bucket-list check mark that could land you in a deadly traffic jam at the summit, gasping for air with other bucket-list check-markers. It's not a peak experience to potentially die waiting in line, so chuck it!

When you gather your friends together to create a chuck-it list, you'll be striking off two of Bronnie Ware's top five regrets of the dying: not being true to yourself and wishing you had spent more time with friends. Depending on what you're chucking, you may also cross off the other top three regrets identified by Ware: working too hard, not expressing your feelings, and not allowing yourself to be happier.

To kick off the "chucking," write out what you will no longer feel compelled to do in each of the following areas. Take about five minutes per category:

· work and finances
· relationships
· health and wellness
· home
· yourself

After each five-minute reflection, share your thoughts with your friends. There may be some chuck-its on your friends' lists that you will want to add to your own. Once you've worked through all five categories, select your top three chuck-its, share them with each other, and commit to holding one another accountable.

Here are a few examples to put you in a chucking mood. Despite a deep admiration for polyglots, Deb stopped "should-ing" all over herself and chucked the idea of learning another language because "it's just too darn hard." She also scrapped gardening after acknowledging she never felt a calming effect from pulling weeds. Julie jettisoned doing the proverbial "thing that scares you most" because she was tired of waking up in a cold sweat. Given that she doesn't like to sweat, she also gave the old heave-ho to running. Lynne, however, did keep running but ditched the idea of completing the Boston Marathon, along with performing any feats of culinary magic that require more than a single pot.

Now it's your turn to come up with a list of things you no longer feel compelled to do. When you're finished, make a toast with your friends to living a life true to yourselves with a glass of the official chuck-it list wine: Trader Joe's Two-Buck Chuck. (Unless, of course, "I will no longer drink cheap wine" is on your list...)

Brag Queens

FROM YOUR GIRL SCOUT BADGE COLLECTION TO YOUR NOBEL PEACE PRIZE, CELEBRATE!

"That brain of mine is something more
than merely mortal; as time will show."
ADA LOVELACE

DO YOU THINK you know your friends' proudest moments and biggest accomplishments? Imagine your surprise if you discovered that one of your friends studied Rhesus monkeys on the island of Cayo Santiago (also known as "Monkey Island") off the east coast of Puerto Rico. That's what we found out about our friend Pam when she became a Brag Queen. Pam loves animals and planned to follow in the footsteps of her idol, Jane Goodall, the English primatologist and anthropologist who is considered to be the world's leading expert on chimpanzees.

Goodall, with her keen anthropological eye, would notice that the activity Brag Queens is the opposite of the chimpanzee dominance rituals she observed in the wild. Chimps throw rocks at their rivals to appear bigger and stronger, but being a Brag Queen is about celebrating the best of one another, throwing roses at each other, so that in the end *everyone* feels bigger and stronger. Being proud of your accomplishments, talking about them, and encouraging others to do likewise are habits worth cultivating.

Many women resist highlighting their achievements because "bragging" has negative connotations. When a woman points out her accomplishments she's often seen as aggressive, while in a similar scenario our male counterparts are more likely to be perceived as confident. It's no wonder that many women in today's workforce struggle with finding an appropriate way to be recognized for their success. Catalyst, a leading global non-profit dedicated to the advancement of women in the workplace, advises that the most powerful tactic for women to move forward in their careers is to simply make their achievements known. Annie McKee, author of *How to Be Happy at Work*, suggests drawing up a list of recent successes to jog your manager's memory of your good work. "Most managers are happy to have that list," she says. McKee goes on to say that another surefire way to get your work noticed is, paradoxically, "to praise and appreciate others."

Let's begin the cycle of appreciation here and praise a few women who have been overlooked in their careers.

Did you know that women were the pioneers of coding and computer programming? If not, you're not alone, as women have been largely written out of its history. The stereotype of women being attentive to details made them the perfect candidates to program the first computers, so from the Second World War until the mid-sixties, the largest trained technical workforce of the computing industry consisted of mostly women. Coincidentally, Ada Lovelace, the daughter of poet Lord Byron and an accomplished mathematician of the nineteenth century, is considered by many to be the world's first programmer.

Ada Lovelace Day is observed internationally on the second Tuesday of October—and is the unofficial Brag Queens holiday—during which women in science, technology, engineering, and math are encouraged to celebrate their successes.

Computer scientist, mathematician, and Navy Admiral Grace Hopper was instrumental in the development of COBOL ("COmmon Business-Oriented Language"), the most successful programming language for business applications in history. Hopper believed that programs should be written in a language closer to English and was said to have coined the terms "bug" and "de-bug" as they relate to the bane of all computer programs. Admiral Hopper was the first woman to be an individual recipient of America's highest technology award, the National Medal of Technology.

Like Grace Hopper, Margaret Hamilton was a computer pioneer and only twenty-two years old when she coined the term "software engineering." Hamilton went on to develop the navigation system used in the Apollo 11 space shuttle that was celebrated in the movie *Hidden Figures*. If it weren't for Margaret Hamilton, who designed the system's software to *prioritize* rather than run operations *sequentially*, Apollo 11 astronauts would have likely aborted the landing on the moon because of a systems overload. It wasn't until 2016, forty-seven years later, that President Barack Obama awarded Hamilton the Presidential Medal of Freedom, the highest civilian award in the United States. And almost as impressively, a year later she became one of LEGO's "Women of NASA" minifigures.

Let's make recognizing each other's accomplishments a part of *our* programming. With the changing era and renewed efforts to focus on equality, it's time for women to put the spotlight on the achievements of which they are most proud.

Brag Queens is an activity that allows you to share your accomplishments with your friends and shamelessly celebrate your collective successes. Reliving your wins and celebrating your friends' achievements creates fertile ground for the seeds of future successes and even greater accomplishments. Whether big or small, all wins born out of your passionate pursuit of excellence made you into who you are today.

There are five steps to this activity:

1 Individually, write out a list of twenty-five brags on index cards.

2 Select ten of them to share with your friends.

3 Cut out each accomplishment and place your cards into a Brag Queen bowl. Mix well. Add glitter. (Not!)

4 Take turns drawing a card—if you draw your own card, throw it back in the Brag Queen bowl—and reading the accomplishment out loud, then attempt to match the brag with its queen.

5 Keep all twenty-five brags and review them often.

The friend with the most correct matches is proclaimed Brag Queen and now has a royal title to add to her brag list! After revealing one another's accomplishments, it's time for you to elaborate on a few brags: select your top three achievements and describe them to your friends without holding anything back, explaining why they are your favorites. Studio audience, don't hold your applause!

Now, at the risk of appearing like aggressive women, we'd like you to join us for a quick Brag Queen procession in which the authors shamelessly boast about their successes.

Of all Julie's achievements, which include earning a CPA designation and a long career in accounting, she is most proud to have raised her three children into responsible and happy adults. Julie is also proud of herself for having the courage to choose time with her family over a coveted senior position at a multinational company because she knew that to be happy she had to live a life she loves.

Deb is proud to have trained and run a marathon at age forty-eight, and perhaps even more so for committing to the eight months of rigorous training beforehand. On the December morning of her marathon on Kiawah Island, South Carolina, she had to arrive at the start line two hours early in subfreezing temperatures. With only a blanket to keep her warm, Deb huddled on the ground with the other runners trying their best not to freeze. Despite the cold, the connection she felt to like-minded strangers warmed her heart throughout the race. And afterward, because she had a free afternoon, Deb capped off the day with a round of golf. Take that, Tiger.

Lynne, a confirmed introvert, is proud of facing her fear (more accurately, *terror*) of public speaking. She took to the stage for six minutes and twenty-three seconds of stand-up comedy at the Absolute Comedy club in Toronto, she was the "Vagina of Ceremonies" in a fundraising production of the *Vagina Monologues*, and most recently she appeared on Toronto's *Breakfast Television* to promote wellness in the workplace. Her Brag Queen mantra comes from writer Anaïs Nin, who once said, "Life shrinks or expands in proportion to one's courage."

We challenge you to find the courage and stamina to totally brag yourselves out. No accomplishment is too small, leave nothing uncelebrated. When the brags are complete, applaud each other and commit to doing something special together to commemorate your combined successes. Try a spa treatment, nature walk, dinner out, or anything you consider to be celebratory.

Taking time to be a Brag Queen will leave you feeling energized, inspired, and motivated to take on your next challenge.

As for our friend Pam, she still admires Jane Goodall and is still an animal lover, but she realized pretty quickly that sweating it out in the jungle with mosquitos and creepy-crawly insects while waiting for chimpanzees to do something noteworthy was not a good fit for her. So Pam moved on to the next chapter of her life and studied law, where she encountered a jungle of another kind ...

A Senseless Dinner

SAVOR A MINDFUL
DINING EXPERIENCE

"Every moment nature is serving fresh
dishes with the items of happiness. It
is our choice to recognize and taste it."

AMIT RAY

SET YOUR PHONE'S timer and close your eyes for a full minute. It's okay, we'll still be here when you get back...

What did you notice? Did the sounds that usually fade into
the background suddenly jump to the foreground? Did you
notice a strange taste in your mouth, a smell coming from an
open window, or a tingling in your toes? Would you volun-
tarily give up your sense of sight for a couple of hours in order
to amplify your senses of hearing, smell, touch, and taste? A
Senseless Dinner is a shared meal during which you turn off
one of your main senses—sight or hearing—so that you can
savor the sense of taste, which we often neglect as we rush
through our days scarfing and swilling.

A heaping plate of evidence suggests that people lacking one faculty begin to use the others more efficiently. If one sense is lost, the areas of the brain normally devoted to handling that sensory information get rewired and put to work processing, supporting, and augmenting the other senses, a phenomenon known as "cross-modal neuroplasticity." ("Neuro" relating to the nervous system and "plasticity" meaning changeable.) This explains how people who are visually impaired, for example, are able to isolate sounds with greater precision and have the ability to experience food in a way the rest of us usually don't.

In Paris in 1997, Frenchman Michel Reilhac and his partner, radio host Julien Prunet, who is blind, opened the first "dark dining" restaurant called Le goût du noir, or "the taste of black." They were inspired by the notion that we take in most of our sensory information about the world visually, yet we experience food through our taste buds. Reilhac wanted to enhance the dining experience by turning off the lights. For some patrons, the lack of vision was an exercise in frustration—hopefully Reilhac and Prunet didn't torment their guests with peas!—but for many others, dining in the dark made them more conscious of the nuances of taste. It must have been a positive sensory experience for the most part, because the concept of dining in the dark quickly spread around the world. In North America, the O.Noir restaurants in Toronto and Montreal and BLACKOUT Dining in the Dark in Las Vegas are examples of establishments where you can experience eating dinner in the pitch black. From BLACKOUT's website: "When the sense of touch, hearing, taste, and smell are heightened, food, drinks, and dinner conversation become a brand new adventure." In other words, without your ability to see, your experience becomes much more conscious.

If turning out the lights seems daunting and you don't want to wear bibs or potentially chase tiny vegetables in the dark, consider dining in silence as an alternative. According to research on eating behavior, dining without conversation, music, or other noise also changes the way you experience food. First, you are more in-tune with what, and how much, you're eating. Conversation is a huge distraction, which is why when we're with friends we tend to eat more than when we're alone. Second, without surrounding noise, you'll be able to hear your food. Yes, food talks in crunches and swooshes that signal freshness, which is why many people love loud, crunchy food—except perhaps when the crunch is coming from someone else.

Inspired by the silent breakfasts he enjoyed at a monastery in India, Brooklyn restaurateur Nicholas Nauman opened a restaurant called Eat and served forty-dollar, four-course dinners in ninety minutes of total silence. "We wanted to bring attention to the physical and visceral properties of eating, and less of the distractions you see so much these days," said Nauman of his soundless dinner. As people settled into the silence, they not only appreciated the subtleties of their food, but they also discovered a latent talent for pantomime with their friends and an overwhelming desire to laugh.

Whatever sense you decide to turn off, A Senseless Dinner is a great place to begin the practice of mindful eating. Mindfulness means focusing on the present moment without judgment. Mindful eating is about being aware of not only *what* you eat, but *how* you eat. It's about fully engaging with the food as you eat it, savoring the taste, and reflecting on how it nourishes your body. Mindful eating reduces stress, improves digestion, and makes you feel more grateful for your food. It can also lead to weight management as you eliminate mindless binge eating and take control of your diet. In the book *Savor*, Buddhist spiritual leader Thich Nhat Hanh and his co-author, nutritionist Lilian Cheung, suggest that "as you become more aware of your body and of the feelings, thoughts, and realities that pre-vent you from taking health-enhancing actions, you will realize what you need to do individually and what types of community and social support you need in order to change your behavior."

You don't necessarily have to turn off the lights or silence the conversation to experience mindful eating. Susan Albers, author of *Eating Mindfully*, suggests other ways to slow down the process, such as using utensils that aren't customary to you, perhaps chopsticks instead of a fork or vice versa. This will force you to take smaller portions, eat more slowly, and look at your food more closely. Other strategies include eating with your non-dominant hand, chewing your food thirty to fifty times per bite, or making your meal last twenty minutes.

As an appetizer to A Senseless Dinner, warm up your mind-fulness muscle with a single raisin. If you don't have a box of raisins in your pantry, you might find a raisin hidden inside some trail mix or raisin bran cereal, or buried deep inside a bran muffin. Examine the raisin and ponder its journey from the grapevine to your hand—it could have easily taken a dif-ferent path and landed in your wine glass instead. Look at the raisin's color and wrinkly texture. Sniff it. Now place the raisin in your mouth and note its sweetness. Chew this raisin *slowly* and as many times as possible. Notice the way it sticks to your teeth before you swallow it and the subtle popping sound it makes when your teeth and the raisin become unstuck.

Share your experience with your friends. What feelings came up? Did this make you anxious? What lessons did you discover by slowly savoring this tiny, shriveled fruit?

Having mindfully eaten a raisin, it's time to expand the experience into A Senseless Dinner and make mindful eating an intentional part of your life. You need never again experi-ence the bitter disappointment of "The Amazing Disappearing Lemon Tart" where you find yourself with sticky fingers and no recollection of what happened to your dessert.

As mindfulness guru Jon Kabat-Zinn says in his book *Coming to Our Senses*, "When we taste with attention, even the simplest foods provide a universe of sensory experience, awakening us to them." And Thich Nhat Hanh puts it like this in his book *How to Eat*: "If we're not mindful, it's not tea that we're drinking but our own illusions and afflictions. If the tea becomes real, we become real. When we are able to truly meet the tea, at that very moment we are truly alive."

Open your eyes to the benefits of savoring life's moments as they occur. And whenever you sit down for a meal, try to remember: there is, in that moment, only food.

5

A Journal of Discovery

VOYAGE TO THE INTERIOR

"I want to write, but more than that, I want to bring out all kinds of things that lie buried deep in my heart."
ANNE FRANK

DO YOU KNOW that writing can ease your pain? Research reported in the *Journal of the American Medical Association* found that people who suffered from asthma and rheumatoid arthritis experienced significant improvement in their health due to the stress-reducing effects of expressive writing—a fancy term for writing from the heart. Popping the cork on pent-up emotions and spilling them onto the page is a great way to rid yourself of their power to hurt you both mentally *and* physically. So gather together for A Journal of Discovery, the activity through which you begin the soulful habit of a lifetime: journaling.

There are many ways to use a journal: to chronicle the day's events and emotions; to capture ideas, dreams, and goals; or to work out problems. But why write it down? Writing is how we give our thoughts substance. Letting a thought ricochet through your mind like a pinball doesn't give you the opportunity to examine it in a productive way. A journal forces you to look at your life with clarity, objectivity, and a sense of possibility.

Reviewing your journal's contents is equally as important as the act of journaling itself. If you review your journal at the end of the week or the month and find the pages filled with the repetitive complaints or reports of activities that accomplish nothing and enable avoidance, it may motivate you to open a fresh page and do some problem solving (see The Power of Twenty, Act 20, if you'd like to journal with your friends on a flip chart). And it is harder to ignore a goal you commit to on paper.

Journaling can turn leaden emotions into golden actions, so who better to share this alchemy with than your friends? Before you get together, encourage everyone to buy a journal. Purchase the most beautiful one you can find, a book that mirrors the importance of its contents and its power to reflect and create a life. If you're inspired, decorate the cover with photographs, headlines, and quotes that position your journal in space and time. And, if your budget allows, buy a beautiful writing instrument that beckons you to pick it up and pour out your thoughts.

Together with your friends, contemplate the blank pages in front of you. And with your pens poised in mid-air, select a theme for your first journal entry. Here are a few options:

- **Problem solve.** Use your journal to write about a current dilemma and hash out alternative solutions.

- **Ask Ellen.** Try out the scientifically proven technique called "self-distancing," where you write as if you were another person giving yourself advice. It doesn't have to be

Ellen DeGeneres. Imagine you're anyone you think would give you solid advice as you record their words of wisdom transmitted to you via your journal.

- **Diarize.** Write about your day, its highlights and lowlights.

- **Dream.** Write about places you'd like to visit, people you'd like to meet, things you'd like to do.

- **Pray.** Write out a prayer of thanks for all that you have in your life, or a prayer asking for guidance.

- **Journal about journaling.** Put to paper the commitment you're willing to make to journaling. What kind of journaling would you like to do? What do you hope to get out of it?

- **Note three good things.** Record three things that went well in the previous week. And, most importantly, share *why* they went well. What did you do right to invite such positivity into your life? (Tip: sharing three good things is the perfect way to kick off any get-together.)

- **"Julia Cameron" it.** Julia Cameron is an author and creator of the practice of "Morning Pages," three pages of uncensored writing where you write out whatever's on your mind, no matter how trivial, bizarre, or socially unacceptable. "I don't know what to write . . . I don't know what to write . . ." is a valid Morning Pages entry that will eventually loosen into reams of what's *really* on your mind.

- **Keep a one-line journal.** For the minimalist, or for those hesitant to make a full-on commitment to journaling, the one-line journal is perfect. Write one sentence that sums up your day. That's it.

- **Use prompts.** Keep it simple by letting someone else write the first few words in your journal entry:

- My favorite childhood memory is...

- The best day of my life was...

- If I could change one thing about myself, it would be...

- An event that changed my life forever is...

- Someone just made me ruler of the world. Here's what I'm going to do...

Don't write as if you expect to submit your journal entry to someone who will give it a grade. The value of journaling is *getting your thoughts on paper* without embellishment. Your journal isn't the place to work on metaphors and clever turns of phrase (although they may appear effortlessly). Spend twenty minutes journaling with your friends, followed by a discussion about what flowed out of the journaling experience. Were there any surprises? We hope so.

If you would like more information, writing prompts, and tips about journal writing, check out James W. Pennebaker's classic book *Expressive Writing*, details of which are included in our Resources section at the back of this book.

6

Childhood Excavations

TAKE A TRIP BACK IN TIME
AND MEET LITTLE YOU

"A grown-up is a child with layers on."
WOODY HARRELSON

IMAGINE THAT YOU suddenly became an amnesiac and lost all of your memories. Who would you be and how would you be able to envision the person you could become? Research suggests that our memories of the past are intimately linked to our ability to create a stable identity and to imagine the future. Donna Rose Addis of the University of Toronto is an expert in the cognitive neuroscience of memory and aging. She studies how autobiographical memory—your recollection of events and information from your past—affects your sense of self and your ability to visualize your future. Addis found that when people with Alzheimer's disease lose autobiographical memory, they also lose a sense of self and the ability to imagine a "possible self." It's like forecasting: the greater number of data points you have from the past, the easier it is to make an accurate prediction. You need the nuggets of your personal history to point you in the direction of your brightest future.

Childhood memories give us insight into who we were, who we are, and who we might become, but trying to retrieve those memories can be like digging for an ancient lost civilization—in quicksand. Yet sifting through your distant past is an excavation well worth undertaking. Discovering lost pieces of yourself is fun and exhilarating and can be the raw material for life-changing decisions.

If you dare to try Childhood Excavations, you'll have to do some digging. Before your next get-together, be sure to visit the appropriate archaeological sites and uncover as many artifacts as possible, including:

- school report cards;

- school photos, preferably class pictures so your friends can have fun trying to pick you out;

- old family photos;

- school yearbooks, hopefully with autographs and cheesy comments;

- music you liked, celebrities you admired, hobbies you engaged in, sports you played.

Childhood Excavations is an activity where you take turns sharing impressionable moments from your childhood and, in the process, become acquainted with who each of you were as little girls. To ensure that your presentations flow like a fast-paced museum tour, you may want to allot an agreed-upon amount of time per friend, and then take turns sharing your tidbits from childhood. Each presenter describes the little girl she was by answering questions like:

- What were her favorite subjects?
- What did she excel in?
- What did the teachers say about her?
- What clubs did she belong to?
- Was she an introvert or an extrovert?
- What was she considered most likely to become?
- Can you glean any clues about who she was from the yearbook messages her classmates wrote to her?

Friends can participate by asking questions to help the sharer uncover long-forgotten truths about herself and her life as a child. Pass your photos around and describe memories of your favorite toys and pastimes. Flip through your yearbooks. Read your report cards out loud.

Before meeting up to participate in this activity, it might be fun to interview some of the people who knew you as a child. What were their impressions of you? You might learn, as Deb did, that she had a flair for event planning—as a child she organized neighborhood fashion shows and led an impressive pot-and-pan parade. Clearly a budding leader, Deb was disheartened to hear a cousin describe her childhood self as "accommodating," but her friends assured her that her accommodation had blossomed into the leadership quality known as empathy.

While The Dinner of Truth (Act 37) is meant to uncover any unfortunate disconnect between who you think you are today and how others perceive you, Childhood Excavations examines the differences that you uncover between "Grown-up You" and "Little You," and is sure to be informative, entertaining, and perhaps even astonishing.

Your Little You has tantalizing secrets that can help you unearth your best life *now*. Once everyone has had an opportunity to share her past, take out a journal and jot down answers to the following questions:

- If Little You could talk to Grown-up You today, what would she say?

- Would Little You be surprised at how she turned out? Would she be proud?

- Would Little You recognize Grown-up You?

The goal of your excavation is to get back inside that little girl's head and find out if you've remained true to what excited her or veered off in an entirely different direction.

All of this exploration could conjure up an "aha" moment, a discovery that you want to reclaim something you once held dear that is missing from your life today. Excavation is important, but the analysis you perform on your artifacts is even more vital. You may have forgotten that you loved French in school and get inspired to take a language course. Through an analysis of her report cards, Julie, who never thought she was athletic, discovered that her eighth-grade teacher said she excelled in sports. Julie's childhood excavations changed the way she thought about herself as an adult. Invite your friends to chime in if they observe something about your past that they think you need to pay attention to.

Once you've thoroughly exercised your memory muscle and relived Little You, choose one forgotten element from your past that will bring more pleasure or fulfillment into your present. If you listen closely, you'll hear the advice of Future You whispering, "*Don't hold back.*"

I Am From

EXPRESS THE POETIC
SOUL OF YOUR UNIQUENESS

"For what is a poem but a hazardous attempt
at self-understanding: it is the deepest part of
autobiography."

ROBERT PENN WARREN

YOUR BRAIN RESPONDS to poetry in a unique and slow-building fashion, just as it anticipates the unwrapping of a gift. When we listen to or read poetry, we can sense when an emotional payoff is coming, and the feeling is intensely pleasurable. Believe it or not, the National Association for Poetry Therapy has a mission to build an evidence-based foundation for the use of poetry as medicine. But we don't need brain scans or advocacy organizations to tell us why poetry has persisted throughout human history: it survives because we need it. As poet Ralph Angel puts it, "Poetry has always existed and will always exist because there will always be the need to say that which cannot be said."

Given that poetry is so powerful, why aren't more people drawn to it? Perhaps it's because we've been taught that poets are tricksters who throw together difficult words, mind-bending metaphors, and opaque symbols just to confuse and intimidate us. Why don't poets simply say what they mean? Why must they obscure the meaning of the poem in such a way that it's available only to those who are skilled in the poetic arts?

Why can't I understand this poem?

Don't be intimidated. Poetry is not the literary equivalent to an escape room, and you don't need to decipher an elusive code to find the only way out: give in to a poem's supernatural mystery and experience each moment as it feels right to you. Poetry makes meaning in the symbolism of dreams—as Adrienne Rich noted in *Arts of the Possible*, "Poems are like dreams: in them you put what you don't know you know." So give in to the dream as you drift into a poetic state of mind, a state of relaxed expectation. As poet Matthew Zapruder describes it in *Why Poetry*, "A poem is like a person. The more you know someone, the more you realize there is always something more to know and understand."

I Am From is an activity that turns a person into a poem. Poets pay attention to the world, become awestruck, and share what they've seen. Pay attention to yourself, become awestruck, and tell your friends about *you*. I Am From will encourage you to think about something that perhaps you have given little conscious thought to until now: how you became the person you are. It sounds daunting, but don't fret. Writing an autobiographical poem is easier and more enjoyable than you think. You don't have to structure it with a strict rhyming scheme like a Petrarchan sonnet (unless you want to increase the level of difficulty). Free verse is what we recommend, the type of poetry with no rules. You can do whatever you want.

In a letter to a publisher friend, poet Robert Frost wrote, "A complete poem is one where the emotion has found its thought and the thought has found the words." Forget about trying to create a perfect poem and aim for the complete poem that resonates with you. What influenced you? How were you raised? What did your parents teach you? What did you learn from your childhood that helps explain your personality and your beliefs as an adult? What was your daily life like when you were a child and how did it make you who you are today? Jot down the first thoughts that pop into your head in response to these questions and get creative.

Writing your poem can be as simple as starting each line with "I am from…" and repeatedly filling in that blank. You don't need to begin each line this way, or even use those words at all, but those who fear a blank page may appreciate having three words they don't have to dream up.

I Am From involves listening hard to the soul and, therefore, is an activity that you may want to begin in solitude *before* your friendly get-together, or you can write your poem while you're surrounded by friends—it's up to you. Even if you decide to write your poems in advance, share them with one another by reading them out loud when you meet. Make it an event, like the coffee shop poetry readings of the beatnik era, with a barstool, candles, incense, and poetic clothing (whatever poetic clothing means to you).

Has a poem ever clicked for you in a way that made you want to read it over and over and over again? If you want to make the evening pack a poetic punch, recite a few of your favorite poems from other poets first. Explain why these mean so much to you. (If you're looking for the perfect poem to read out loud, check out our Resources section for a few of our favorite suggestions.)

Whatever you do, park your digital devices at the door of your poetry extravaganza, because one of the main benefits of poetry is that it forces your mind to detach from the pull of the everyday and drift in an entirely different direction.

Smartphone notifications have a nasty way of spoiling the state of wonder that a poem can create. Poetry also forces you to slow down. You can't rush through a poem, scarfing its contents like an email swallowed whole while in the express checkout line at the grocery store. A poem is meant to be savored, its words read carefully, so that you can adjust to its rhythm, melody, harmony, and strangeness. Generous, open yet focused attention is the most important quality you can bring to a poem. And to one another.

It's an honor to listen to an I Am From poem, an invitation into the poet's deepest thoughts. Listening to a poem is an act of empathy, as we think along with the poet and reflect on our common humanity. Through writing and sharing your poem, you will enrich your relationship with your friends, but more importantly, you will connect deeply with yourself.

Where are *you* from?

Here's a sample of an I Am From poem by Deb, to get your poetic juices flowing:

I am from family values and family visits.
I am from Dad's work ethic
And Mom's optimism.
I am from "Do your best" and "Do your homework"
I am from appreciating life's little pleasures.
New adventures,
New challenges,
And trying new things.
I am from The Golden Rule ("Do unto others...")
Respect for self
And respect for others.
I am from love for self, family, and life.

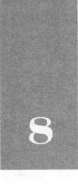

Moments of Meditation

DON'T JUST DO
SOMETHING—SIT THERE!

"Meditation connects you with your soul, and this connection gives you access to your intuition, your heartfelt
desires, your integrity, and the inspiration to create a
life you love."

SARAH MCLEAN

IT'S OUR HOPE that two activities from this book will become
regular agenda items for your get-togethers: Move Ya Body (Act
34), a physical workout; and Moments of Meditation, a workout for your mind. Previously considered a hippie pastime, and
now practiced by CEOs, entertainers, and athletes, meditation
involves quieting the mind, often by turning your attention to a
single point of reference, typically either the breath or a single
word or phrase known as a mantra.

This mental workout has more benefits than you may
realize. Harvard researcher Sara Lazar has been using MRI
technology to determine the effects of meditation on the

brain. Her study results suggest that meditation can alter the brain in several areas. Lazar found that in the part of the prefrontal cortex associated with memory and decision-making, fifty-year-old meditators had the same brain thickness as twenty-five-year-old non-meditators. In another study of people who enrolled in an eight-week course in meditation, regions of the brain associated with learning and compassion became denser, but the amygdala (the fight-or-flight area of the brain) shrunk, indicating that subjects had trained themselves to become less reactive to stress.

Meditation might sound easy, but anyone who has tried to meditate knows that the untrained mind resists all attempts to tame it. The Buddhist term for this is "monkey mind," meaning a restless, unsettled, uncontrollable mind. Considering we have roughly 3,000 thoughts per hour, it's no wonder we have difficulty controlling them. Our minds swing from one thought to the next without much consideration. We swim in our thoughts without realizing how lost we are in them, like the proverbial fish who responded to the greeting, "Morning, boys, how's the water?" with "Water? What the hell is water?" But when we stop for a moment and hit the pause button on life to meditate, we realize that there is something beyond our thoughts. An objective observer inside each of us can free us from the belief that we are our thoughts and help us to realize that our lives are made up of endless possibilities.

For this act of friendship, you will practice meditation together during a friend date. The benefits of Moments of Meditation will be felt in just a few minutes as your brains ride alpha waves to relaxation. We prefer the term "shared meditation" versus the more common "group meditation" because something special happens when you *share* this practice with your friends. Through shared meditation we experience our own calmed state, but we also participate in each other's sense of peace and compassion thanks to the phenomenon known as "emotional contagion," the idea that we feed off one another's meditation-enhanced moods. When you meditate with your best friends you realize that there's no need for perfection, you're not the only one who repeated the mantra twice before a to-do list popped into your head and your monkey mind carried it away to the produce section of the grocery store. Meditating together encourages you to build the habit within an atmosphere of acceptance and belonging. Moments of Meditation will deepen your bonds of friendship as your practice reveals, in the quietest moments, how everything and everyone is connected.

They call it "practicing" meditation because taming the mind is a skill that you can improve with repetition. If you and your friends are new to meditation, start small, with just five minutes, and progress from there. Taming 250 thoughts in five minutes is enough of a challenge for the novice. Meditation typically involves silencing the mind by focusing on a mantra or your breathing. But *guided* meditations are great for beginners—they are like adding training wheels to your meditation practice. Do a Google search for "guided meditations" and you'll find a selection of online resources to download free of charge prior to your next get-together.

There are many different types of meditation, but the one we've repeatedly used is self-compassion meditation, or "metta." Metta involves repeating a mantra (such as "may you be happy, may you be healthy, may you be at peace"), offering these wishes to yourself and then extending them to loved ones, to people you're indifferent toward, to people you actively dislike, and finally, to all of humanity. When incorporated into a meditation practice, self-compassion can become powerful; it can reduce stress and improve social connections and life satisfaction. Kristin Neff offers a number of guided self-compassion meditations at self-compassion.org. And if you'd like to explore other types of guided meditation, Tara Brach offers a wide range of meditations of different lengths and for various purposes on her website, tarabrach.com.

After you complete Moments of Meditation, you may wonder if you did it right. Roger Thomson, a psychologist and a Zen meditator, told *Psychology Today* that there is one way to know: "If you're feeling better at the end, you are probably doing it right."

9

To Give Is to Receive

GO TO THE PLACE WHERE CREATIVITY MEETS GENEROSITY

"Kindness in words creates confidence.
Kindness in thinking creates profoundness.
Kindness in giving creates love."

LAO TZU

WANT TO GET high? We're not talking about drug-induced euphoria, but rather the organic, self-generated endorphin high you experience when you give. A "helper's high" is the elation you feel after the act of giving which lights up the same part of the brain that gets turned on by stimulants like food or sex. Even remembering an act of generosity can create a mini helper's high.

According to "The Social Capital Community Benchmark Survey" conducted in 2000 by researchers from Harvard University, those who gave contributions of time or money were forty-two percent more likely to be happy than those who didn't give. Why do our brains reward us for giving? Altruistic

47

behavior makes sense when we look into our evolutionary past: helping others was critical to the survival of the tribe. One can imagine the offering of food, comfort, or whatever passed as a gift thousands of years ago (a shiny rock?) as a form of social glue that helped to bond people in a circle of giving and receiving.

Today, thanks to the gift of science and research by Scott Bea at the Cleveland Clinic, we know that regular acts of generosity have been linked to the following health benefits:

- lower blood pressure and stress levels;
- increased self-esteem and happiness;
- less depression;
- longer life.

Giving is good for you, which is why we recommend a daily dose of generosity. It doesn't have to cost a thing. A handwritten note, a compliment, a small act of kindness—even smiling at a stranger—all qualify as gifts that spread happiness.

A good way to establish a lifetime habit of generosity is to start with your friends, making gift-giving to them a springboard to a wider circle of generosity. Begin by giving a thoughtful group gift to commemorate a friend's special occasion, or even draw names—secret-Santa style—to give gifts to each other. We've done both, and we have fond memories of giving as a group to an individual and of getting each other presents, just because.

For To Give Is to Receive, try to think way outside the gift box. It's been our experience that the best presents are the ones you've never received before, and will likely never receive again. For one of Deb's "special birthdays," Lynne found an artist, who also painted toenails, to create a masterpiece portrait of us from a collection of our photos. Lynne knew she was in trouble when the artist called her finished work a "caricature." An impressionistic work may have been acceptable, or even an abstract, but a caricature? Milestone birthdays can be challenging enough without someone exaggerating the features you've spent years learning how to camouflage. Lynne was embarrassed, but Deb was a good sport about the rendering—even though it portrayed her as if she were viewed through a wine glass—and proudly hung the caricature in her hallway.

If you decide to give a gift as a group to a single person, start by spending some quiet time alone, thinking about that friend. Ask yourself repeatedly, "What could we do that would make her happy?" Noodle this question individually throughout your day, then get together, share your thoughts, and collectively decide on the perfect gift. It may be the handcrafted result of a beloved hobby, or a favorite movie or book that you want to share. The Power of Twenty (Act 20) is a great way to come up with gift ideas.

A fun spin on individual gift giving involves a trip to the dollar store. Start by drawing names to decide who you'll be buying for. Then, as a group, determine a dollar amount each person is to spend. We recommend ten dollars or less. Keeping the amount low will help your pocketbook and give you better results by forcing you to focus and be creative. The happiness generated by To Give Is to Receive is directly proportionate to the creative thought and personalization put into the gift, not its monetary value. Now plan a group excursion to a dollar store. Try to find something—anything—that represents the personality or essence of the friend you're giving to and that costs roughly the same amount as a couple of fancy coffees.

To keep yourself from mindlessly wandering and inhaling too much of that indescribable dollar store smell, think about your purchase metaphorically. Look for the perfect item that encapsulates the person you're buying for. Let's say you feel that your friend Karen is always juggling balls—or if she just loves the game of tennis—you might choose a container of tennis balls. If you see her as a person with a sense of humor, look for a joke book or a fake nose and glasses to represent her comical side. Is she a caregiver? Perhaps bandages and a can of chicken soup symbolize her strengths for you.

Once you've completed your shopping assignment, it's time to gather and take turns presenting your purchases, along with explanations about what the items represent. Or if you want to increase the level of engagement and ratchet up the enjoyment, mix all of the purchases up and try to match the gift with the friend.

Regardless of whether your gift took ten days or ten minutes to find, whether it was strategically planned or spontaneously mischievous, To Give Is to Receive will leave you feeling calm, positive, and full of gratitude. And doesn't it make sense that a path to a generous life starts with giving a gift to a friend?

10

Mock Therapy

LET YOUR FRIENDS HELP YOU CUT
YOUR PROBLEMS DOWN TO SIZE

"My focus is to forget the pain of life. Forget
the pain, mock the pain, reduce it. And laugh."
JIM CARREY

WHY WRITE TO a syndicated stranger to ask for advice about
the boss who intimidates you, the neighbor who annoys you,
or that special favor your husband asked you to perform last
night, when you have a panel of friends with years of experience, unique perspectives, and a genuine desire to help?

The mock therapy approach we recommend does not
involve an exhaustive Freudian analysis of your childhood or
multiple lengthy counseling sessions. It does, however, require
a sense of humor and a wild imagination. The word "mock" is
derived from the Old French *mocquer*, which may have orig-
inated from the Vulgar Latin *muccare*, meaning to "blow the
nose." In Vulgar Latin times, blowing your nose at someone
was an egregious insult...

"Go and boil your bottoms, sons of a silly person. I blow my nose at *you*, so-called 'Arthur-king,' you and all your silly English knnnniggets!" This is a classic example of Monty Python giving the search for the Holy Grail some mock therapy.

Mock Therapy is in no way blowing its nose at psychotherapy, nor is it intended to be a substitute for professional help. But for situations where your friends can offer a valuable suggestion or strategy, Mock Therapy may be healing.

Taking something that looms large in your mind and giving it a physical form that *mocks* it down to a more reasonable size can defuse tension and give you a new perspective. In Mock Therapy, you take a situation, person, or memory that makes you feel fearful or shameful and tease it into an art or craft.

Mock Therapy consists of three easy steps:

1 Individually decide what you want to parody. It may be an upcoming event, a person, or a memory that fills you with fear or shame, simply intimidates you, or makes you feel uneasy.
2 Now with your friends, imagine different ways you can mock the source of your fear, or shame it through craft or performance art.
3 Create and present or perform the spoof of your problem.

Here's an example: In Mock Therapy, Deb imagined that an acquaintance who intimidated her was the "Golden Girl," so named because everything she touched seemed to turn to gold. She had the best husband, the best clothes, the best job, the best house on the street, and the best way of being the best. This Golden Girl often elicited a feeling of inferiority in Deb, who said, "Around her, I feel like ... a bobblehead." Deb used a golden statuette of a woman dressed in the finest English golf attire (did we mention her acquaintance was also the best golfer?) to represent the Golden Girl and a bikini-clad bobblehead doll to depict herself. As Deb channeled the Golden Girl describing her impressiveness to the group, Lynne and Julie chimed in with absurd lines, exaggerating her total awesomeness and taking her audacity to new egotistical heights, while Deb's bobblehead could only babble and chortle. Everyone had a good laugh and a mocking good time. The next time she saw the Golden Girl and heard more examples of how wonderful her life was, Deb may still have nodded like a bobblehead, but she was laughing on the inside.

No matter if you're Jungian or Freudian, humor is the secret weapon in the Mock Therapy arsenal. The benefits of laughter have been known for centuries; there is a long and successful history of its use in medicine, and recent research supports its links to good health. As an adjunct to therapy, ancient Greek physicians would prescribe a visit to the hall of comedians (the ancient Greek equivalent of a Netflix comedy special) as a key element of healing. And in the fourteenth century, surgeon Henri de Mondeville would use humor to distract his patients from the pain of surgery without an anesthetic. More recently, the study of laughter has been given an academic name, gelotology, and several landmark studies have revealed just how powerful laughter is. Humor can reduce blood pressure and stress hormone levels, ease anxiety and depression, and strengthen the immune system (although laughing is highly contagious). Social laughter has been shown to increase pain tolerance, and the ability to maintain a sense of humor and laugh about your difficulties can act as a positive coping mechanism.

Mock Therapy can take the form of a skit, an opera, a voodoo teddy bear, a crayon caricature, or a rant. It can be anything, as long as it passes the Jim Carrey test: you must laugh while you're in Mock Therapy. Now, gather your friends together and blow your nose at your problems.

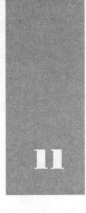

11

Thank You, Thank You, Thank You

COP AN ATTITUDE OF GRATITUDE

"Showing gratitude is one of the simplest yet most powerful things humans can do for each other."
RANDY PAUSCH

THANK YOU, THANK You, Thank You combines two soulful activities: gratitude and writing. All you need to complete this exercise are index cards, thank-you notes—as plain or fancy as you like—a favorite pen, and an attitude of gratitude. Oh, and a gratitude jar—an old-fashioned glass jar with a ribbon tied around it.

You can't travel far along the path of self-development before you encounter gratitude as a cornerstone of emotional wellbeing and achievement. Amit Sood, creator of the Mayo Clinic Resilient Mind program, wrote *The Mayo Clinic Handbook for Happiness: A 4-Step Plan for Resilient Living* and, you guessed it, one of the four steps includes a gratitude practice.

We can all be grateful for the voluminous research on gratitude from which we draw one undeniable conclusion: Thank You, Thank You, Thank You is good for you.

Based on the groundbreaking research of gratitude pioneer Robert Emmons, among others, we know that there are psychological, physical, and social benefits from a gratitude practice, and they include:

- reduced stress, anxiety, and depression;
- increased immune system function;
- increased enthusiasm, optimism, and sense of self-worth;
- improved sleep quality and duration;
- reduced blood pressure;
- better relationships;
- less loneliness and social isolation;
- a shift in focus from the self to others, which is the defining feature of self-transcendence.

Unfortunately, the journey of transcendence through gratitude isn't easy. We all have a built-in negativity bias that was put in place eons ago to ensure our survival: pausing to enjoy a beautiful sunrise and give thanks for the abundance of nature could have turned our ancestors into some creature's breakfast. Therefore it's easier to focus on what's wrong or threatening than to appreciate all of the good that there is. It takes effort to be grateful, so we have compiled three science-based practices to help you reap the benefits of gratitude: gratitude cards, the thank-you note, and the ceremonial gratitude jar.

Begin with an activity inspired by Robert Emmons' research. Everyone gets a stack of index cards—the more the better—and for twenty minutes write down a person, place, object, memory, or event that you're grateful for. One item per card. To get the most gratitude boost from the activity, be specific and describe *why* you're grateful, not simply what you're grateful for. Try to write five complete sentences for each item, because you need to *feel* gratitude to get its benefits, and a shorthand list just won't cut it. Recall and record unexpected experiences, as they seem to elicit a greater gratitude response, and try to focus on people.

Next, go around the room and have everybody read what they've written down, then place their cards in the gratitude jar. By the time you've finished and all of your index cards are in the jar, you should feel thoroughly grateful and ready for the next exercise: the thank-you note.

Gratitude is a relationship-strengthening emotion because it encourages us to be humble and acknowledge our dependence on others. Think about someone who has changed your life for the better and take a few minutes to write a note of thanks to that person. Read your thank-you notes out loud to each other while you mindfully evoke the emotion of gratitude. Be sure to mail your thank-you letters, or better yet, deliver them in person.

Who had the most touching thank-you note? Congratulations! You're the first person to get custody of the ceremonial gratitude jar, guaranteed to brighten any day. Draw a random card from the jar any time you need a pick-me-up, and add to the jar with a fresh index card whenever you feel the urge to express more gratitude. Rotate stewardship of the jar from friend to friend and keep the circle of gratitude going in a continuous cycle of Thank You, Thank You, Thank You.

As common as the advice to be grateful has become, the power of this activity can't be overstated. Keep exercising your gratitude muscle by filling out a weekly gratitude card on which you write down the details of something that went well that week and why. And if you'd like a bonus twist on the gratitude exercise that forces you to focus on the object of thanks, have everyone write a "daily gratitude haiku" for a week. A haiku is a poem of three lines with five syllables on the first line, seven on the second and five on the third.

Here's an example:

It's hot and humid
Why complain when this is a
Winter vacation

At your next get-together, have everyone share a week's worth of gratitude haikus with the most illuminating example of this gratitude art receiving a literary prize, such as a gratitude haiku journal, a beautiful writing instrument, or a tray of sushi.

Take notice of how your gratitude practice affects your life. Do you feel more abundant and positive, less anxious and happier? Are your relationships improving? As thirteenth-century German philosopher and theologian Meister Eckhart put it: "If the only prayer you said in your whole life was, 'Thank you,' that would suffice."

12

Forgive and Hike On

DISCOVER THE ART OF FORGIVENESS, NATURALLY

"To forgive is to set a prisoner free and discover that the prisoner was you."

LEWIS B. SMEDES

AUTHOR JOHANN HARI suffered from depression for his entire adult life. In his book *Lost Connections*, he describes how he, a man who thought Central Park was too rustic, was enticed into climbing a mountain in the Rockies just outside the town of Banff, Alberta, Canada. Researchers say that awe is the natural antidote for anxiety and depression, and Hari experienced it firsthand. Surrounded by nature, he was overcome by a feeling of reverence and the sense that the world is big and our ego and its concerns are small. Hari's mountain guide, evolutionary biologist Isabel Behncke, said, "It's almost like a metaphor for belonging in a grander system," referring to the freedom and perspective that we get when we immerse ourselves in nature.

Hiking and forgiving are a perfect pair. Hiking is a truly awesome way to commune with nature, work your body, and feed your soul's longing to return to its ancient roots. And nothing eases the mind, body, and soul more than forgiveness, which becomes a little easier as the ego shrinks in the presence of nature.

We are healthier when we Forgive and Hike On. According to the Mayo Clinic, forgiveness can lead to:

· healthier relationships;
· less anxiety, stress, and hostility;
· lower blood pressure;
· fewer symptoms of depression;
· a stronger immune system and improved heart health.

There is no better way to rid yourself of the weight of negative emotions than by hiking. The expansiveness of nature begs us to unburden ourselves and to travel lightly. Holding a grudge or harnessing feelings of bitterness or regret can be all-consuming and disruptive, making it challenging to form healthy new relationships or think about anything other than the cause of so much pain.

It may seem punitive and superior to hold a grudge. "I love my grudges. I tend to them like little pets," says Reese Witherspoon's character in the TV series *Big Little Lies*. But as the Buddhist saying goes, "Holding on to anger is like grasping a hot coal with the intent of throwing it at someone else; you are the one who gets burned."

"Holding on to a grudge really is an ineffective strategy for dealing with a life situation that you haven't been able to master," says Frederic Luskin, founder of the Stanford Forgiveness Project. According to Luskin, forgiveness can help to reverse the anger and hopelessness that manifests from the inability to cope with grudges.

Before you put on your hiking boots, write a Declaration of Grudge in which you describe how you feel about the person or hurtful event that you've been burdened with, and why it's not okay. Acknowledge that the pain of harboring a grudge is coming from the hurt feelings, not from the act that birthed the grudge. Describe those feelings. How would it feel to let go of the hurt? Remember, Forgive and Hike On is about making yourself feel better and changing your grievance story to serve you, it's not about anyone else. Once you've described what letting go would feel like, turn your story around. On a separate sheet of paper—your Declaration of Forgiveness—fully express what forgiveness means to you and what benefits you expect to receive once you've forgiven. Take back your power and cast yourself as a hero in your story of forgiveness, stressing what you learned from the experience and how it has made you stronger.

With both declarations in hand, you're ready to get together and Forgive and Hike On. It doesn't matter if your path to forgiveness is along an established hiking trail or a well-traveled dirt path close to home, as long as you're immersed in nature and you walk far enough that you feel physically removed from your everyday life.

Take turns working through the following four steps:

1 **Express your grudge.** Read your grudge document out loud to your friends, or if you aren't comfortable sharing what you've written, read it silently to yourself.

2 **Cultivate empathy.** Put yourself in the offending person's hiking boots and consider all possible reasons for the hurtful act. What were their intentions? How might they perceive the same incident? Have you made a similar mistake in the past? If you're sharing with friends, ask for their thoughts.

3 **Look at the positive.** Read your forgiveness document out loud, sharing the benefits of what happened to you and

reminding yourself that forgiveness is about personal power, the heroic choice to forgive. Negative events rarely travel alone or happen to just one person, so for a minute or two dwell on these silver linings and compare notes, because it's likely your friends have had similar experiences.

4 **Symbolically let go.** Express your forgiveness for the person or the act out loud, rip up your Declaration of Grudge, and bury it. Or eat it. Your choice. Eating your grudges— use edible wafer paper and edible ink—is both cathartic and environmentally friendly.

Once you've all completed the exercise, if the experience has moved you and you feel so inclined, join hands with your friends and say a quick prayer of thanks before continuing on your hike. Do you feel a bit lighter having traveled the path to forgiveness? You should. You just lost the burden of carrying around negative feelings.

Forgive and Hike On was a powerful experience for the three of us—far more so than we had anticipated. It was definitely not the activity we had the most fun with, but it was certainly one of the most rewarding. This act of friendship strengthened our bond, and nature reminded us that grudges are *not* like little pets that should be loved and tended to, as in *Big Little Lies*, but instead are varmints that should be released into the wild.

It's Easy Being Green

IS YOUR CARBON FOOTPRINT TWO SIZES TOO BIG?

"There is hope if people will begin to awaken that spiritual part of themselves, that heartfelt knowledge that we are caretakers of this planet."
BROOKE MEDICINE EAGLE

IT ISN'T EASY being green if you're Kermit the Frog. With their jelly-like unshelled eggs, frogs are extremely vulnerable to climate change. Imagine Costa Rican Kermit sitting on a mountain watching little froglets die because global warming has raised cloud levels and his offspring are now exposed to a harsh, dry environment. He can move up the mountain to a place where it's cooler, but it's also more crowded. Eventually Kermit, like the rest of us, will reach the peak of the mountain, and there will be nowhere else to go.

Climate change is arguably *the* most important issue of our time. Consider these facts from NASA: In 1950 carbon dioxide levels surpassed the highest levels they'd ever been, and they continue to rise at an unprecedented rate. Most climate scientists believe that the warming of the planet is due to humans. The earth's temperature has increased almost two degrees Fahrenheit since the late nineteenth century, with the five warmest years occurring since 2010. Our oceans are warming and our glaciers are in retreat. Visit NASA's Global Climate Change site for more facts and check out the video of Swedish teen activist Greta Thunberg, who put climate negotiators in the hot seat during the United Nations climate summit in December 2018 in Poland.

There are countless ways we can take better care of our beloved Earth. Even though sometimes it feels like the problems are too big and complex, and that we're just one person in seven billion who can't possibly make a difference, we all must take action to save our planet for future generations. So gather together for this critical activity of developing your group Paris Accord—an "It's Easy Being Green Accord," in which you state, item by item, what you can commit to do to address climate change.

Here are a few ideas to get you started: Use energy-efficient light bulbs and programmable thermostats. Turn off the lights whenever they're not needed. Clean clothes with energy-efficient appliances and hang them to dry instead of using a dryer. Use a dishwasher rather than handwashing. Try steam cleaning rather than using toxic chemicals. Carry reusable bags, mugs, and cutlery. Stop purchasing bottled water and other single-use plastics. Put a time limit on showers. Cut down on or eliminate air travel. Carpool, take public transit, and ride a bike. Consume more Local Roots (see Act 35) and eat less meat. Cows, pigs, sheep, and goats are responsible for significant methane emissions, a global fart that is far worse for the environment than carbon dioxide.

There are a few additional items you might want to consider adding to your accord that aren't as familiar as reducing your meat consumption to help lower harmful cow emissions. Consider hanging on to your smartphone for as long as possible. Researchers James Suckling and Jacquetta Lee determined that the production of a single iPhone 6 released 178 pounds of carbon dioxide into the atmosphere. And fast fashion isn't green—it's better to buy high-quality clothes and keep them for a long time or buy secondhand. A high-quality wardrobe is something we can all rally around. Finally, don't waste food— it's been estimated that about forty percent of food in the United States is thrown away.

We challenge you to put ten items on your It's Easy Being Green Accord (or whatever you decide to call it), plus commit to at least one *collective* action that will reduce your carbon footprints before everyone signs it. Plant a tree or trees (tree planting is one of the best strategies to fight climate change), visit a local farmers' market, make your next shopping expedition to a vintage or consignment store, or have an organic cleaning products party where you make your own household cleansers out of vinegar, lemon, and baking soda. These are just a few examples of how friends can go green together.

It's Easy Being Green because we all need to.

As Greta Thunberg says, "I want you to act as if your house is on fire. Because it is."

A Friendly
Multiple-Choice Quiz

IF YOU'RE NOT SURE HOW WELL
YOU KNOW EACH OTHER, PICK C

"Isn't life a collection of weird quizzes
with no answers to half the questions?"
PAWAN MISHRA

HOW WELL DO you know your friends? How well do they know you? If you've been friends for ten years or more, you may think you know one another extremely well, but do your friends know that you once played the part of a mosquito in an ice carnival (Lynne), that you purchased a yellow angora sweater with the proceeds from your first job (Julie), or that your first (but not last) spanking came at the hand of a neighbor lady who caught you bolting into the middle of the street (Deb)?

If you think that asking questions about each other makes you "nosy parkers," then think again. The Mayo Clinic endorses the benefits of friendships and suggests that one way to nurture relationships is to open up to your friends, adding that friendships provide a sense of belonging, improve self-confidence, promote overall health, and reduce stress.

The reward-to-effort ratio for A Friendly Multiple-Choice Quiz is remarkably high, even without factoring in the Mayo Clinic's findings. Each friend simply writes ten multiple-choice questions about herself that she thinks none of her friends will know the answers to, and when you get together, you see which friend gets the most right. You may be surprised to discover that writing the questions is most of the fun, and don't be offended if four out of ten is the highest mark anyone gets.

For the best results, prepare your ten questions and circulate them before you meet so everyone has time to consider their answers. When you have your get-together, read each question out loud, allowing each person an opportunity to announce her answer and the rationale behind her choice before you give the correct response. As with quiz shows with returning guests, you may find that you'll want another round of ten questions—and then another—before crowning the champion who knows her friends best.

We had so much fun when we did A Friendly Multiple-Choice Quiz. It was strangely exhilarating to share obscure personal information and make a couple of outrageously wrong guesses. Most of the questions that stumped us were from the prepubescent and teenage periods of our lives, which is not too surprising given that our friendships began much later on.

Here are a few sample questions to inspire you.

1 When Lynne was a little girl, she had a stuffed animal that she enjoyed kissing, nibbling, and throwing up on, which, as it turns out, was great practice for marriage. She named her animal:

(a) Mr. Cuddlesworth
(b) Pookie

(c) Booboo
(d) Wally
(e) Mr. Man

2 In grade school, Deb had to attend a special class for a slight disability. That disability was:

(a) Attention-Deficit/Hyperactivity Disorder
(b) Speech Sound Disorder
(c) Dyslexia
(d) Stuttering
(e) Severe shyness

3 Julie was teased at school because:

(a) She wore glasses
(b) Her ears stuck out
(c) She had freckles
(d) She had two yellow teeth
(e) She had no friends

A Friendly Multiple-Choice Quiz can be as casual or as personal as you're willing to go. Whether your questions are profound or ridiculous, your friendships will grow stronger and you'll find some weird reasons to stay friends. If you're curious to know the answers to our friendly quiz, here they are. Lynne: (e). Lynne's mother became so concerned about Lynne's profound attachment to the threadbare blob known as Mr. Man that she hid him behind a kitchen canister. Deb: (b). Speech Sound Disorder. Her r's sounded like w's. Weally! Julie: (d). She fell down the stairs, knocked out two baby teeth, and the adult ones grew in a different color. Happy to say they were eventually replaced with white ones.

15

A Woman's Rite

CELEBRATE THE DIVINE
IN ALL THAT'S FEMININE

"Through the Goddess, we can discover
our strength, enlighten our minds, own
our bodies, and celebrate our emotions."
STARHAWK

CAN YOU IMAGINE what early humans thought about the act
of giving birth? Thousands of years before ultrasounds, sex ed
classes, and father of eight Mick Jagger cynically singing
about how newborn babies happen every day, it's possible that
humanity looked at birth as the miracle that it is and believed
that women possessed extraordinary creative powers that mir-
rored the magic of the natural world.

Could goddess worship be the oldest of the old-time
religions? Scholars studying ancient societies have found evidence of goddess worship in the curvy carvings that have been
unearthed, but there is much speculation about whether the
abundance of womanly shapes in archaeological findings is

suggestive of goddess worship, or simply prehistoric pornography. It would make sense, however, that primitive societies who depended on the abundance of the earth, the breeding of domestic animals, and the fertility of the tribe would also value the female form as a powerful symbol of survival.

There is evidence that supports the existence of ancient societies where women were in charge, cultures that flourished for thousands of years and generally lived in peace with hamlets that lacked defensive fortifications and funeral customs where men and women appeared to have had equal status. The aim of these matriarchal cultures was not for women to have absolute power over others but to embrace maternal values that honored the cycles of nature and nurtured the power within.

The suppression of goddess worship in Europe is believed to have occurred a few thousand years before Christ, when the Indo-Europeans invaded Europe from the East, bringing with them the emblems of modern civilization—war, belief in male gods, exploitation of nature, and knowledge of the male role in procreation. Goddess worship didn't totally disappear, but it became subordinate to the devotion to male gods among the Greeks, Romans, and Celts. Women could no longer exist as equal partners in civilizations founded on brute strength, and so "herstory" became history.

It's empowering to imagine cultures in which women were revered, and it's in this spirit of prideful femininity that we propose you resurrect the old goddess culture for one charmed evening. "You know when I feel inwardly beautiful?" Jennifer Aniston once asked. "When I am with my girlfriends and we are having a goddess circle." This act of friendship is a celebration of the sacred feminine with A Woman's Rite, to honor the feminine aspects of the universe as well as our female ancestors. The purpose is to take a few minutes to reflect on the power of the sacred feminine. What is it about being a woman that gives you joy? What is it about the women in your life that makes you love them?

For A Woman's Rite goddess circle, each friend brings a few items that she feels represents a particular woman or aspect of womanhood that she wishes to honor. These can be used to decorate an altar with symbols of femininity. Lilies, papayas, and shells are all potential altar ornaments. Candles for each participant, ceremonial bread and wine, music, and mementos of the women who have shaped your life will create a warm, feminine atmosphere.

Holding hands and expressing thanks is a good place to begin. The following is a sample gratitude script you might recite, but it's far better if you repeat words you have written yourself:

Women who have paved the way before us
We thank you
Women who devoted their lives to causes that eliminate suffering
We thank you
Women who give selflessly to others
We thank you
Women who speak their truth even as their voices shake
We thank you
Women who help others heal and grow
We thank you

To all the women who have come before and to those who made a difference in our lives today, we thank you for that which you have ignited within us. We promise to pass on the flame of feminine strength and wisdom.

You may want to light candles sequentially and include a reading. Maya Angelou's poem "Phenomenal Woman" is a great choice. You can also drink ceremonial wine and talk about the women who inspire you and the items you brought with you to commemorate these special women.

We have suggested an agenda, but A Woman's Rite can be anything you want it to be. It doesn't have to be serious. You could sacrifice SPANX or any other symbol of twenty-first-century femininity that you find oppressive: skinny jeans, diet soda, fashion magazines, anti-wrinkle cream, mascara, pantyhose... you get the idea.

When we did A Woman's Rite, Lynne shared her admiration for Nobel Prize–winning author Alice Munro, Julie invoked the Goddess Oprah, and Deb shared the life story of her maternal grandmother, Mary Gertrude Stadler Hiatt. During the Great Depression, while raising eight children who were close in age, Mary seemed to have a never-ending supply of breast milk, and even breastfed babies from the local orphanage. In the midst of this, Mary took over her husband's custodial position at the neighborhood church when he became fully paralyzed from muscular dystrophy. She took great care of her bedridden husband, ironing his sheets so he wouldn't get bedsores. Mary had a great intellect and a wicked sense of humor. She was a woman everyone adored and a goddess in her own right. Do you have women in your life like Deb's grandmother or famous women who you admire and would like to celebrate?

Take some time with your friends to acknowledge the feminine energy in the universe. It's not only inspiring, it's a woman's right.

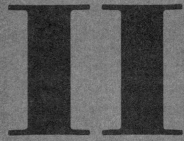

II

acts of creativity

"There is a fountain of youth:
it is your mind, your talents, the
creativity you bring to your life and
the lives of the people you love."

SOPHIA LOREN

16

Think on Your Stilettos

IF YOU CAN SPEAK ABOUT NOTHING, YOU CAN TALK YOUR WAY OUT OF ANYTHING

"It usually takes me more than three weeks
to prepare a good impromptu speech."

MARK TWAIN

think on your stilettos • *figurative*
To be able to speak coherently on a random topic while balancing on long, thin high heels for an audience of friends (*we were awestruck by her ability to think on her stilettos as she expounded on the ins and outs of envelopes*).

CAN YOU TALK for a full minute without interruption on the subject of rubber bands? Many people, especially introverts, don't consider themselves capable of speaking extemporaneously (the fancy word for thinking on your stilettos), because often in conversations the perfect line doesn't come to them until twenty minutes after the opportune moment has passed. But learning to Think on Your Stilettos is a skill like any other, and has more to do with the confidence that comes from doing it well in an accepting environment surrounded by friends than with innate talent. Introverts, who prefer to ponder for several minutes or hours before they open their mouths, will particularly benefit from Think on Your Stilettos because they will find it exquisitely painful. At least at first.

You may never have to regale an audience on the elastic subject of rubber bands, but chances are, at some point in your life, all eyes will turn to you, and you will be asked to share your thoughts. Will the thoughts tumble out like plastic monkeys from a barrel, leaving your audience dazed and confused by the tangled mess, or will your listeners be awed and enlightened by your oratorical gifts?

Comedian Jerry Seinfeld has joked that our fear of speaking is so severe that at a funeral, most of us would rather be the person in the casket than the one standing behind the podium delivering the eulogy. We hope that Think on Your Stilettos will help you become so comfortable with ad-lib public speaking that you'll consider trying International Extemp, the bungee jump of public speaking, an event where speakers from around the world compete on their ability to prepare a seven-minute current-events speech in thirty minutes.

You may think that verbal fluency isn't critical, and that you can coast through life without ever being called on to make a toast, but when sociologist Andrew Zekeri asked college graduates which skills were most useful in the business world, oral communication ranked number one. Public speaking helps develop critical thinking as well as verbal and non-verbal communication, and the more you practice public speaking the less afraid you will be when asked to say a few words.

Think on Your Stilettos starts with everyone writing a single word on a slip of paper and folding it up and putting it in a bowl. The more common the word, the better, like pineapple, toothpick, calendar, or soap. Mix up the papers in the bowl and choose someone to make the first pick. All they have to do is speak for one minute about the word they draw. Sounds simple, doesn't it? The problem is that we are accustomed to setting our own verbal agendas, and the to-and-fro of conversation gives us a breather once we've run out of things to say.

To perform a monologue on a random topic is a skill rarely, if ever, used. But it's a great way to keep your brain nimble and ready for conversational surprises or encounters with (other) introverts, when you have a lot of empty conversational space to fill.

A variation of Think on Your Stilettos is to scan your sur-roundings for an object to talk about for a full minute. Try to convince your friends that the object is meant for some purpose other than what it's known for.

Let's use a clothespin as the object. It could be described as a "chip clip" to keep the bag of chips closed, but that's a fairly common use for clothespins. To dial up the creativity, one might hold up the clothespin and announce in a confident voice that the object is a "gloves pincher," a gadget used by women during the Victorian era to keep their gloves handy when they weren't wearing them. They would pinch their gloves together and then fasten the pincher to their handbag or the side of their boot. Another item that might be repurposed is a melon ball scoop. This could be described as an instrument used by ophthalmologists in the eighteenth century to examine their patients' eyes by looking through the hole in the center of the scoop. (You thought we were going to say scoop their eyeballs out, didn't you?)

These ideas should not be judged on feasibility but rather applauded for originality, humor, and the passion of the friend who is presenting. Be sure to applaud the fledgling efforts of the introverts in your group in proportion to the redness of their cheeks, and give your friend with the most unique explanation something ingenious as a prize. Deb made an impassioned presentation in which she inflated a rubber kitchen glove and convinced us that it was used to cure people with a fear of hands, narrowly beating Julie whose CPA designation added credibility to her assertion that the gloves were used by accountants to handle dirty money, and Lynne who said they were used for clown burlesque. For her creative efforts, Deb won a bottle of Mamma Mia! Pizza Beer.

Think on Your Stilettos hones your ability to speak concisely and with clarity. It exercises your brain's creativity and imagination, too, which can in turn help with everyday problem-solving and decision-making. And, if you feel you would benefit from remedial Think On Your Stilettos training, choose a few words and do one-minute monologues alone in your car or join Toastmasters, where Think on Your Stilettos is called "Table Talk."

Get On Board

LET YOUR FRIENDS HELP YOU
MAKE YOUR DREAMS COME TRUE

"I guess these visualizations really, really work."

BIANCA ANDREESCU

WHAT DO JIM Carrey, Arnold Schwarzenegger, Oprah Winfrey, Tiger Woods, and 2019 U.S. Open tennis champ Bianca Andreescu have in common? Other than being famous, they've all used visualization to manifest what they want and who they want to be. Although visualization has a whiff of woo-woo, there are scientific studies that suggest using the power of imagination can help to bring about a desired reality.

A Cleveland Clinic study entitled "From Mental Power to Muscle Power—Gaining Strength by Using the Mind" demonstrated the power of the mind-body connection when groups that were doing only mental training increased their muscle activation without performing the physical activity. Okay, it was just finger and elbow strength, but it's something. Similar studies, which compare athletes performing physical activities with those who only visualize them, show that mental practice alone can improve performance. There are tangible physical results when we use the power of our minds to imagine what we want to have happen, and visualization makes it more likely that we'll notice opportunities in support of our goals, opportunities that we might otherwise miss.

Get On Board is an activity where you visualize who you want to be, what you want to have or do, and capture it in a form that will engage your subconscious mind, trigger emotions, and inspire action. The friendly twist in Get On Board is that, instead of designing your own vision board, you brief one of your friends, who then creates it for you. This board will become the prompt for your brain to be on the lookout for opportunities to turn your vision into reality. Having a friend design your board for you has two main benefits: first, she will be more objective about your goal and will be able to create something more realistic; and second, your friend will be able to focus on the journey rather than be captivated by the rewards.

According to research, a drawback of vision boards that focus on the end result is that the brain relaxes, perceiving that the goal has already been attained. When you ask your friend to Get On Board, make sure she captures not only what you desire but also how you will get there. For instance, if you want to run a marathon, the board should show the sweat and grind that goes into training. If you want to be a bestselling author, the board should include a picture of you pounding the keyboard and attending events. Have at least as many scenes that depict your path to success as you have visions of reaching your goal, because how you get there is as important as the end point.

Get On Board will require some advance preparation. You'll need to spend time on the visioning part so you'll know what to tell your friend to reflect on your board. Everyone will need to brief her partner on her goal. Your vision board can be focused on work, relationships, self-image, family—wherever you'd like to see change in your life. Make sure it's a goal that excites and motivates you to do whatever it takes to get there. The partners can be selected either randomly, or strategically by selecting a friend with some expertise in the area you want to excel in.

To translate your friend's mental images into physical form, you'll need a poster board, scissors, glue, a selection of colored markers, inspirational quotes, and images from magazines or the Internet. Use whatever it takes to depict her vision and create the emotion that will inspire her to action. For best results, choose a simple, uncluttered message. You'll be surprised at how quickly and organically the images and text come together, as if you were putting together the pieces of a puzzle that already exists rather than composing from scratch.

Once everybody has completed their vision boards, present them to their owners. Because they are gifts from friends, the boards will be imbued with magical properties. Take a photo of your board so that you can shrink it down to postcard size and make multiple copies. Keep them by your bedside, stick one on your bathroom mirror, or make it the wallpaper on your phone so you get a boost of inspiration every time you look at your screen (if you're the average person, this would be about sixty times a day).

Regardless of how you choose to remind yourself of your vision, Get On Board has the power to transport you and transform your life. And remember: it all began with a friend.

18

Carefree Karaoke

BECAUSE SINGING SUMMONS SEROTONIN

"If everyone started off the day singing,
just think how happy they'd be."
LAUREN MYRACLE

COULD IT BE that human history began as a musical? Perhaps not an Andrew Lloyd Webber musical—although it's fun to imagine a Neanderthal production of *Cats*—but some historians believe humans sang before they started talking. The idea that language came from song feels right, doesn't it? Charles Darwin also believed that the origin of language was song and he imagined our ancestors serenading each other with love ballads.

So when did we lose our singing voices?

Daniel J. Levitin, psychology professor at McGill University and author of *This Is Your Brain on Music,* believes we stopped singing about five hundred years ago when the first concert halls appeared in Europe. He explains that "the audience was meant to sit with their hands politely folded in their laps and their mouths shut" while performers sang onstage. Singing was something that specialists did while others watched. Over time, the distinction between professional singers and everyone else resulted in a fear of singing in public. Other than in houses of worship, the only place many of us break out in song is either in the shower or in the car. Sadly, even a round of "Happy Birthday" in a casual family environment can sound half-hearted at best.

It's unfortunate that so many people shy away from singing—convinced that if they can't be Adele, they won't even try to carry a tune—because singing is beneficial to our health and wellbeing. Singing reduces stress, helps us communicate, and encourages cooperation. Even more than that, singing is exhilarating.

Neurological research has found that our brains release oxytocin when we sing, and an even bigger dose when we sing with others. Oxytocin, known as the "love hormone," is a chemical involved in social bonding that fosters togetherness. Levels of oxytocin increase when we kiss or hug someone, and play a huge role in sex, birth, and breastfeeding. Besides prompting a surge in oxytocin, singing in groups releases two other powerful hormones: dopamine and serotonin. Dopamine activates the brain's pleasure center and serotonin reduces anxiety. And if that isn't enough, singing makes you breathe deeply without thinking about it, naturally relaxing you.

Group singing magnifies the physical and psychological benefits of song, and can strengthen an entire community. A global study of over 1,700 choir members found that women benefit physically, socially, and emotionally from singing significantly more than men, and both sexes enjoy the way it increases social connection and cognitive stimulation.

The amplified benefits of group singing are enticing some companies to introduce choirs into the workplace as a wellness activity that not only boosts employee health, but also promotes teamwork and improves productivity. As reported by Cassie Werber in *Quartz*, one such company is Triodos, a bank in Bristol, England, where employees gather once a week to sing in the lunchroom. Triodos' chief operations officer, Judy Rose, said that although singing takes people out of their comfort zone, once they've made the leap, it helps build self-assurance, adding it "gives confidence, a feeling of achievement—and fun." And there are studies that support Judy's claim. Claudia Röhlen at Rhine-Waal University of Applied Sciences in Germany studied the power of ensemble singing and found that participants in workplace choirs felt a sense of interconnectedness, an effect that brought them both relaxation and euphoria. Group singers also experienced joy, confidence, and gratitude, Röhlen says, feeding into an overall experience of "self-transcendence"—a sense of going beyond their own ego and feeling like they're part of something greater.

Are you ready to transcend your ego and join your besties in song? Carefree Karaoke is designed for friends to sing together and connect with the ancient communal joy of song in a non-threatening setting, without the pressure of a panel of judges. It's carefree because our version of karaoke is not the kind of singing where you might regret what you sang the next day (as Lynne regretted singing a song with the line, "I will go down with this ship" on a cruise); rather, it's singing along with your friends which can help eliminate any self-consciousness you might feel about the quality of your voice. You don't need a karaoke machine. All you need is a little help from your friends. If you still have doubts about whether you can sing without a glass of wine, try Carefree Karaoke while you're on a hike or road trip with your friends. There's something about facing the same direction with limited eye contact that takes the pressure off.

There are three simple steps to this activity:

1 Before your next get-together, have everyone select three of their favorite songs to sing along to, and inform the friend with an Apple Music, Spotify, or similar music subscription service to add them to your Carefree Karaoke playlist.

2 Print off the lyrics and bring them with you, or find a link on the Internet with the lyrics to share with your friends.

3 Put your Carefree Karaoke playlist on shuffle, play your songs at full blast, and sing like no one's listening. Because they aren't.

Podcast host Bobby Bones selected his "Top 5 Car Sing-Along Songs," which we hope will serve as inspiration: Queen's "Bohemian Rhapsody," Bon Jovi's "Livin' on a Prayer," Neil Diamond's "Sweet Caroline," ABBA's "Dancing Queen," and Journey's "Don't Stop Believin'."

Whether it's on a hike, a road trip, or a get-together where the urge to sing overcomes you and your friends, Carefree Karaoke will release the hormones that encouraged our ancestors to belt it out. Lynne and Deb were thrilled to discover they both knew all the words to The Eagles' "Lyin' Eyes," and both Lynne and Julie were in awe of Deb's savant-like ability to repeat the first line of almost any song, based on only a few seconds of its intro. No matter if your singing voice is sultry torch singer, perky pop vocalist, or roaring rocker chick, find it and start singing! Who knows, Carefree Karaoke might become your favorite way to harmonize with your friends.

19

Mud Pie on Your Face

BEAUTY NEVER TASTED SO GOOD!

"Beauty begins the moment you decide to be yourself."
COCO CHANEL

BACK IN SIXTEENTH-CENTURY Europe, having pale skin that was untouched by the sun was considered a sign of beauty, wealth, and power. To create a pale appearance, a mixture of white lead and vinegar called Venetian ceruse was applied to the face, neck, and chest. It was most famously used by Queen Elizabeth I, and not only did it make the skin "grey and shriveled," but in some cases it also resulted in a death mask caused by lead poisoning. Amazingly, Venetian ceruse remained popular for more than three hundred years in spite of its side effects, which also included hair loss, mental deterioration, and muscle paralysis.

By the end of the nineteenth century, a desire for more natural, youthful-looking skin led to a new variety of beauty products, such as Madame Rowley's Toilet Mask. An ad for this pliable, rubber, overnight mask read, "recommended to ladies for Beautifying, Bleaching, and Preserving the Complexion." The product didn't stay in favor for long after people found it suffocated the face, encouraged perspiration, and frightened family members. As science marched to the forefront of society, several beauty treatments were offered in an experimental spirit, including raw meat facials, radium-laced beauty products, and freckle removal with nitrogen. The endless search continues for a magical concoction we can slather on our faces that will make us glow (hopefully not in a radioactive fashion like radium did). The latest candidate? Cannabis-infused cosmetics.

As an act of rebellion against the random beauty standards that have enslaved women for centuries, and against the toxic products sold in the name of beauty, gather together with your friends and create a pop-up spa where you apply to your faces something non-poisonous that is guaranteed to make you look delicious. We call this activity Mud Pie on Your Face because we concocted a face mask made of the tastiest thing we could think of: chocolate.

For ninety percent of its history, an estimated three to four thousand years, chocolate was consumed as a beverage. The word "chocolate" comes from the Aztec word *xocolatl* meaning "bitter water." Chocolate has long enjoyed social, religious, and monetary significance, with both the Mayans and Aztecs believing it had magical, even divine, powers. When the Spanish added sweetener in the form of cane sugar or honey, chocolate became popular in Europe. The Italian adventurer and author Casanova was said to be especially fond of drinking chocolate, which was believed to have nutritional, medicinal, and aphrodisiacal properties.

Chocolate lovers like Casanova would have enjoyed a mud pie facial, the edible chocolate treatment that's guaranteed to put on a happy face. Packed with antioxidants to fight skin-damaging free radicals, our mud pie serum is a hydrating face mask for regenerating and restoring your skin with instant results. And it comes with mood-elevating whiffs of chocolate. It is just one of dozens of do-it-yourself treatments you can apply with ease.

Here's the recipe for our favorite chocolate facial mask, but if you're allergic to chocolate, or would like to try a different ingredient, then explore the Internet for recipes using kefir (probiotics such as kefir or Greek yogurt offer your skin a bath in friendly bacteria), bananas, avocadoes, or anything else you'd love to dip your face in. If you can't be bothered to prepare a Mud Pie on Your Face do-it-yourself mask, just slap on some Nutella.

Mud Pie on Your Face

Ingredients:

- one tablespoon of pure cocoa powder (antioxidant)
- one tablespoon of sour cream (moisturizer)
- four teaspoons of honey (antibacterial, anti-inflammatory, and deep pore cleanser)
- one teaspoon of ground oatmeal (gentle exfoliant)

Directions:

1 Combine all ingredients in a bowl.
2 Apply mixture liberally to face.
3 Leave in place for ten to twenty minutes or for however long you can resist eating it, then rinse with warm water.

Caution: fits of laughter will cause cracks in your chocolate face mask. This will result in flaking that is positively delicious.

Don't hide the camera for this exercise. A lot of the fun of Mud Pie on Your Face (aside from eating the product) comes from defying the Instagram filter—the Venetian ceruse of the twenty-first century—and the notion that a woman must be perfect before she can be seen on social media. Just remember the most important rule of beauty according to Tina Fey: "Who cares?"

20

The Power of Twenty

RIDE OUT A BRAINSTORM AND GET A RAINBOW OF FRESH IDEAS

"If coming up with ten ideas sounds too hard, then come up with twenty."
JAMES ALTUCHER

IN 1938 EXECUTIVE Alex Osborn, the "O" in BBDO advertising agency, whose clients included General Electric, Chrysler, and Goodyear, had a problem: a lack of fresh new ideas for his company's ad campaigns. Alex turned to a four-hundred-year-old Hindu technique called *Prai-Barshana* (*Prai* meaning "outside yourself" and *Barshana* meaning "question"), in which a problem is stated in a simple, specific way, and solutions are generated in a group setting, without judgment. Criticism, eye rolling, and head shaking are strictly prohibited, although participants are allowed to build on a suggestion. Osborn called the process "brainstorming." Not, as you might suspect, because it causes the painful sensation of a raging storm inside the head, but because it uses the brain to "storm" a problem.

The Power of Twenty is a simple yet effective activity that will harness the collective mind power of your friends, and use it to storm a challenge in need of ideas. We may not be trying to dream up new ideas for ad campaigns, but everyone faces challenges for which there are multiple possible solutions. To begin, the person facing the challenge provides a short background of the problem she's trying to solve, summarizing the need for ideas by writing "Twenty Ideas to..." with the "..." being an area of her life that's stuck. For example, she might write "Twenty Ideas to Market My Business," "Twenty Ideas to Fundraise," or, if she's brave, "Twenty Ideas to Improve My Life." Number a piece of paper from one to twenty (if you have a flip chart handy, as we often do, that would be ideal) and start brainstorming as a group. Write down the ideas as they come, without judgment.

At first, the ideas will flow quickly and you might struggle to keep up with writing them down, but after the low-hanging fruit has been plucked, you may find it difficult to reach higher levels of creativity. When that happens, take a break and talk about something else, anything else, as far removed from the subject at hand as possible. In his book *Hyperfocus*, author Chris Bailey calls letting your attention wander "scatterfocus." It turns out that letting your mind go is a great way to generate ideas without trying. Knitting (see Close-Knit Friends, Act 32) is one of Chris Bailey's favorite ways of letting idea generation miraculously happen.

Here are a few more pointers for idea generation:

- Pretend to be someone who you admire, and generate ideas from her (or his) perspective.

- Imagine the stupidest idea you can cook up. Freeing yourself from the pressure of generating good ideas gives ingenuity room to flourish.

- Thumb through magazines or browse the Internet in search of images that nudge your creative right brain.

- Pick a random word from the dictionary and try to tie ideas to it. For example, if you're looking for ideas to improve your love life, the word "Brazil" might give you the idea to take samba lessons or play a Bebel Gilberto soundtrack in the bedroom or get a Brazilian wax.

- Think big! What idea would put you on the evening news?

Some ideas will seem obvious, others will seem odd, but at least a few will contain seeds of brilliance. Creativity sometimes flows in spurts, often piggybacking on a previous thought, and you'll find that the suggestions improve as the group warms up. By the end of the activity, we guarantee that you'll have twenty more ideas than you had before you started The Power of Twenty. After you fill in the twentieth blank, you may want to have a celebration, but make it brief because now comes the tricky part: the presenter must *act* on one of the ideas immediately, even if it's just finding a phone number, in order to take one small step toward her goal. This activity is so easy and effective that someone in your group may want to begin another The Power of Twenty challenge right away.

In his blog, hedge fund manager, entrepreneur, and author James Altucher describes how important it is to exercise your "idea muscle," which will atrophy just like any other muscle when you're not using it. Instead of waiting until you're forced to come up with ideas, Altucher advises everyone to "strengthen that connection to that idea force inside of you" now. He goes on to say that by writing down at least ten ideas a day for six months, you'll become an "Idea Machine," and, as you continue this practice, "your life will change every six months."

The more ideas you generate in your life, the better your decisions will become. Imagine what twenty suggestions can do, especially when you keep exercising that generative-idea muscle, following through on at least something on the list, so that the ideas that came from your inner worlds can appear in the outer world.

Helen Keller once said, "Ideas without action are worthless." So don't waste The Power of Twenty.

21

Dances with Bellies

SHAKE YOUR HIPS WITH YOUR INNER GODDESS

"Belly dancing is the way for the body to smile."
SOHEIR ZAKI

ACCORDING TO PETER Lovatt, a dance psychologist at the University of Hertfordshire in Britain who is also known as "Dr. Dance," movement changes the way we think. In an interview with *The Guardian*, Dr. Dance said, "We know that when people engage in improvised kinds of dance [such as belly dance] it helps them with divergent thinking—where there's multiple answers to a problem." You may therefore want to combine the creativity-enhancing Dances with Bellies with our brainstorming activity The Power of Twenty (Act 20).

Through his research, Lovatt has found that dance can be used as therapy for people with Parkinson's disease, a condition known to disrupt the divergent thinking process. Other studies have shown that dance can relieve symptoms of depression, boost your mood, and improve self-confidence. Dance has even been used to help traumatized people express what can't be spoken, to connect with others, and to release tension. We're all rhythmic beings: our hearts beat, our brains pulse, and our bodies are governed by circadian rhythms. When we tap into our own natural cadence through dance, something wonderful happens.

Belly dancing, known in scientific circles as "solo-improvised dance based on torso articulation," is an ancient and thoroughly feminine mode of bodily expression. Not just for the belly or the stomach, belly dancing involves the hips, the legs, and most especially the arms and hands (surprisingly, good arm work is what distinguishes the most skilled belly dancers). The faster you move, the greater the cardiovascular workout, but it's your sensuous spirit that belly dancing stimulates most intensely. We're most accustomed to dancing in steps, moving back and forth in a horizontal direction, but the belly dance is a largely vertical dance of the core muscles with bare feet connected to the ground.

There are many theories about the origins of this most earthy dance, often referred to as "the world's oldest dance." Some believe that belly dancing began more than six thousand years ago in pagan fertility cults as a ritual dance for fecundity and childbirth. "If you opened the dictionary and searched for the meaning of a Goddess, you would find the reflection of a dancing lady," wrote Sufi poet Shah Asad Rizvi, and it's believed that the first belly dances were performed by priestesses as invocations to a female deity.

One of the most appealing aspects of Dances with Bellies is that there are no body shape or age restrictions, and participating in this fluid and erotic communal dance draws out the goddess in each of us. Some aficionados will tell you that the best belly dancers are over forty because belly dance is about sharing love, life experience, and self-acceptance. Regardless of the age of the dancer, the belly dance is a passionate, and sometimes defiant, celebration of female sexuality. Prominent belly dancer A'isha Azar calls the artform "a rebellion wrapped in a flirtation." When you dance with your belly, the goal is to feel the language of your body so completely that you forget you're a dancer and become the dance.

To take the first steps in becoming the dance, put on a pair of yoga pants or a long skirt, and wrap a colorful scarf around your hips to encourage you to move your pelvis freely. If you have a belly dance supply store handy—and who doesn't?—consider purchasing a pair of finger cymbals or a coin belt so that you jingle whenever you move. A coin belt or scarf, symbolic of the coins the belly dancer would receive in payment for her artistry, is an instant conversation piece at any party or a sparkling accessory for your next corporate presentation, especially if you've mastered the hip snap that adds *oomph* to any message. A sports bra or bathing suit top completes your belly dance costume, leaving bare your tummy, which is the focus of the dance. Unfortunately many women—particularly those who have given birth (Julie's one)—are self-conscious about their bellies. Dances with Bellies encourages you to show your midsection some love, and give it the spotlight it deserves.

It's easy to belly dance the Dances with Bellies way: you simply follow Shakira's instructions and dance with hips that don't lie. There's no need to learn hip drops or infinity loops or earthquake shimmies. Simply feel the music with your whole body and use it as a form of self-expression.

Gather in a circle for some "shared rhythmic torso articulation," connecting visually and physically with your friends as you dance. Cue a belly dance playlist (all music streaming services have them) and let your bellies loose as everyone contributes movement ideas. Take turns dancing in the middle of the circle and encouraging one another's bellies. Don't be surprised if laughter erupts, massaging your tummy from the inside.

It's our hope that Dances with Bellies makes you feel joyful, beautiful, and empowered. Now go, and dance with the goddesses within.

22

Change Your Clothes, Change Your Life

WHAT IS YOUR WARDROBE SAYING BEHIND YOUR BACK?

"You can have anything you want in life if you dress for it."

EDITH HEAD

HAVE YOU EVER changed your clothes from something extremely casual, like athleisure or pajamas, to a formal ensemble and suddenly felt like an entirely different, more sophisticated person? Well we have, and there's a name for this phenomenon: "enclothed cognition." A study out of Columbia University and California State University entitled "The Cognitive Consequences of Formal Clothing" found that dressing in more formal clothes than your friends, classmates, or co-workers tends to make you think more abstractly, holistically, and creatively.

William James, the father of American psychology, put a tremendous emphasis on clothing, placing it just after the physical body, and before immediate family, when he described the essential elements of the self. The body is the site and clothes the materials with which we, the architects of our wardrobe, build the person we are.

James understood that clothing sends a message to the world *and* to ourselves, and considering how to dress should be a thoughtful decision. But most people follow along with the crowd and let the fashionistas decide what they will wear. William James was drawn to unfashionable polka-dot ties, a signal of self-awareness and deliberate nonconformity at a time in the late nineteenth century when men were instructed to be "self-forgetful" and blend in. His lectures at Harvard were picturesque, and so was his colorful, casual, idiosyncratic style. James dressed to display the qualities he valued: approachability, creativity, and openness. He consciously chose his clothing to affect how he felt about himself, because he knew his feelings would influence his behavior.

We change our clothing and our clothing alters us, giving us an emotional boost or accentuating feelings of depression. What's the go-to depressing wardrobe item? According to a survey conducted by Karen J. Pine of the University of Hertfordshire in Britain, we're most likely to throw on a pair of jeans when we're feeling blue. Pair these with a baggy top, and—voilà!—you've got the perfect depressing ensemble. As Jerry Seinfeld said to George Costanza on "The Pilot" episode of *Seinfeld* when he saw his hapless friend decked out in sweatpants, "You're telling the world: I give up. I'm miserable, so I might as well be comfortable." If she were alive today, Coco Chanel would be leading the charge against sweatpants and sweatshirts, as per her timeless advice, "Dress shabbily and they remember the dress; dress impeccably and they remember the woman."

Coco's pearls of wisdom aside, what does your outfit say to *you*? German researchers who asked people to describe their character traits when they were dressed in casual clothes were more likely to describe themselves as "easy-going" or "clumsy," versus "neat" or "strategic" when they were formally dressed. It's not frivolous to think about your choice of outfit as a reflection of your state of mind. As Pine reports in her book *Mind What You Wear*, sudden changes in outward appearance have been associated with mental illness. Depressed people often lose interest in clothes, preferring to dress down, fade out, and blend into the background rather than stand out.

Pine believes that by changing your clothes, you can change your life, and more importantly, transform how you feel about it. You dress up your thoughts in your clothes and can't help but slip into the characteristics you associate with certain items of clothing. Put on a stylish hat and you will become the confident person who isn't afraid to attract attention—you're the kind of person who wears a hat.

How do you want to dress up your thoughts? Your friends can help. Change Your Clothes, Change Your Life is a rotating fashion party where, in recurring get-togethers, you visit one another's homes, pour yourselves some champagne (like the supermodels do), and investigate your closets together. But *before* you hit the closets, we highly recommend that you watch Stasia Savasuk's "Dressing for Confidence and Joy," an inspirational TED talk on fashion that's anything but superficial.

Also before you start, answer the following questions in writing and share your responses with your friends so that they can help you create the look for the life you want:

1 What outfit currently in your closet makes you feel like you're on top of your game? What three adjectives would you use to describe this outfit?

2 How would you like other people to describe you when they first meet you?

3 Who are your fashion icons?

4 How do you want your clothes to make you feel?

5 When you imagine your best possible life, where are you and what are you wearing?

Now that you know the look you want, keep in mind that there's a lot of money invested in the contents of our closets. We all know that we tend to reach for the same few items, ignoring clothes with the "clearance sale" tag still dangling like a forgotten Christmas ornament, or items decorated with the dust of neglect. A study of over 18,000 households in over twenty countries by relocation-services company Movinga revealed that Americans wear *only eighteen percent* of their clothing, which means we need our friends to help us get the most value out of our entire wardrobe and to create the look and feeling we want. Friends, your role is to give honest feedback, provide creative ideas for putting new outfits together, and most of all, to ensure that whoever is the host of Change Your Clothes, Change Your Life is sending a purposeful message with her apparel.

The beauty of this act of friendship is that it's not about fashion trends, it's about deciding who you are, what you want to communicate with your attire, and, with the help of your friends, making your unique style happen.

As Virginia Woolf wrote in *Orlando*, a novel in which the protagonist changes their clothes *and* their gender, "Vain trifles as they seem, clothes have, they say, more important offices than to merely keep us warm. They change our view of the world and the world's view of us." Change your clothes, and you can't help but change your life.

23

A Friendly Q&A

EVERYTHING YOU WANTED TO KNOW ABOUT EACH OTHER...

"One key pattern associated with the development of a close relationship among peers is sustained, escalating, reciprocal, personal self-disclosure."

ARTHUR ARON

WELCOME TO THE act of friendship that encourages you to engage in sustained, personal self-disclosure that escalates and is reciprocal. Sound intriguing?

Asking and answering questions is one of our all-time favorite friendly activities. It sounds so simple, yet A Friendly Q&A can be extremely powerful and enjoyable, as researchers discovered when they used a series of personal questions to develop intimacy between strangers.

The thirty-six questions developed by psychologist Arthur Aron and others in his now-famous study "The Experimental Generation of Interpersonal Closeness" has even helped people fall in love. The first couple who pilot-tested the questionnaire fell for each other, got married, and invited Aron and the rest of his lab to the ceremony. But that's not the end of the story. In an essay for the *New York Times* entitled "To Fall in Love with Anyone, Do This," author Mandy Len Catron took Aron's thirty-six questions out on a date. She describes how she and her soon-to-be-boyfriend were like two frogs gradually warming in a pot, the intimacy cranked up just a little bit with each ensuing question until it eventually boiled over into love. Questions are portals to the kind of trust and closeness that deepen relationships, both romantic and platonic.

Questions are also springboards to great conversations. Sherry Turkle, an MIT professor and an expert in interpersonal closeness, advocates for more and better conversations as a way of cultivating empathy. When we are fully present with each other, sharing our experiences of joy and sorrow and making an effort to relate to each other, we are at our most empathic. Turkle calls conversation "the talking cure," and rightly so: don't you feel better when you closely listen to another person and know that you have been heard? (You can practice becoming a better listener with A Night at the Improv, Act 31.)

Before your A Friendly Q&A get-together, write out at least ten questions on slips of paper and label them according to one of three escalating categories: innocent, nosy, or brazen. For example, an innocent question might be "As a child, what was your favorite board game?" A nosy question is "What is something you purchased but wish you hadn't?" A brazen question would be "If your love life were a kitchen gadget, what would it be?" (Our answers, which will remain anonymous: double boiler, spice rack, and crème brûlée torch. Ouch!)

Questions that would seem appropriate for a job interview or those with a negative slant, such as "Name three positive character traits that you do not possess," are highly discouraged. Remember this: if you pose a question, you must also answer it. If you don't have time to dream up your own questions, check the Resources section, which includes a link to Aron's thirty-six questions.

Take turns drawing questions, reading each out loud, and asking the person whose answer you would most like to hear to respond first. Everyone, including the person doing the asking, answers each question. Time will pass enjoyably as the topics bounce around from the sublime to the ridiculous, filling your mind with increasingly illuminating information about each of your friends, drawing you even closer together.

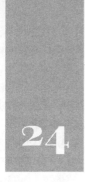

This Playlist Is Me

IF YOU WERE A MUSICAL ANTHOLOGY, WHAT WOULD YOU SOUND LIKE?

"Where words leave off, music begins."
HEINRICH HEINE

BEFORE WE WERE born, we listened to music. Thanks to the pioneering work of South African researcher Sheila Woodward described in Elena Mannes' *The Power of Music*, we know that the womb has its own ambient soundtrack. An underwater microphone that Woodward adapted to safely fit inside a uterus revealed there is a symphony of sound inside the womb, muffled music and conversation, the drum of a heartbeat, the hum of breath. Scientists using MRI technology have found that no part of the brain is untouched by music. Music penetrates our bodies: we can close our eyes, but our ears remain open, taking in music and making it a part of us.

In his song "Trenchtown Rock," Bob Marley sings about how when music hits you, you feel no pain, affirming the healing qualities of music. Researchers have found that music can indeed reduce chronic pain. And because it has such a powerful effect on body and mind, music can help to heal people, such as Congresswoman Gabby Giffords, whose gunshot wound to the brain left her unable to speak. Giffords lost her speaking voice, but she could sing the words she couldn't say and, through song, built a new road back to language. Alzheimer's patients can also benefit from the magic of a song that evokes a particular time and place, recapturing lost memories.

Have you ever wanted to let the power of music speak for you? If so, then This Playlist Is Me is the activity to provide the soundtrack for your next get-together.

There are a few ways to approach your musical monologue:

1 **Make an autobiographical musical poem.** What is the first song you remember? What song reminds you of high school, falling in love for the first time, a memorable trip? Create a chronological playlist of your life, and for each song, write a line or two that explains the meaning behind the music to your friends, the sillier the better. Sample liner notes from Lynne's This Playlist Is Me read: *"I'm Gonna Wash That Man Right Outa My Hair" (Mitzi Gaynor)—When I was a little girl, my mother sang show tunes to me while she washed my hair, and this song, from the musical* South Pacific, *was her favorite. As she sang, I imagined a little man covered in baby shampoo tumbling into the sink.*

2 **Choose a playlist of "Songs That Stick."** The autobiographical musical poem described above consists of songs that mark a time and place—and chances are you won't like these songs anymore, at least not with the same passion they once kindled. Songs That Stick, however, should be a playlist of music that has become part of your soul. These are the songs that sing to you, no matter how many times you've heard them. Have some fun with this and make

the last track your anthem—the song that inspires you the most and reflects your philosophy of life. Now review your playlist and give it a title. In an interview with NPR, singer-songwriter Tom Waits said, "I like beautiful melodies telling you terrible things." Tom's Songs That Stick playlist might therefore be called, "A Beautiful Terrible Playlist."

3 **Create a playlist of the music that is you *right now*.** This playlist is a collection of music that you're into at this moment in time. You may not like Cardi B's latest hit next month or even next week, but for now, it's the music that can uplift you in an instant and help you reach the finish line, even when your gas tank is empty.

Have each friend create one playlist in any category ("autobiographical," "stick," or "right now") on your preferred platform—Spotify, Amazon, Apple Music, and so on—to play at your next get-together. Be sure to explain the rationale behind each song so that, whenever your friends hear it, they'll be reminded of you. Deb and Lynne always think of Julie when they hear "I Am Woman." "Wild Horses" is Deb's song and it's always accompanied by a visual memory we have of her involuntarily racing into the distance, holding tightly to the mane of a wild horse named Joey that was bolting back to its stall.

We know it's totally old school, but if you want to create a memento of this activity, complete with cover art, then burn a CD to turn this activity into "This CD Is Me."

In Jodi Picoult's novel *Sing You Home*, Zoe, the protagonist, is a music therapist who uses music to heal people with mental illness and emotional challenges. In the book Zoe asks, "What songs would be on a mix tape that describes you? ... Seriously," she adds, "if you looked through the Favorites list on my mother's iPad, you could probably sketch her out as thoroughly as if you'd met her in person. This is true of anyone: the music we choose is a clear reflection of who we really are."

After you've listened to the playlist that is one of your friends, try to describe the person behind the choice of music. Were there any surprises? Is it possible to explain why a song speaks to you?

Use the power of music to express the part of you that words leave out.

25

Draw on This

STICK PEOPLE ARE PEOPLE TOO!

"The problem isn't that you can't draw.
It's that you believe you can't draw."
CHRISTINE NISHIYAMA

ARE YOU SOMEONE who thinks that she can barely draw stick people? Well, stick people are drawings, and if you want to see what stick people can do, check out the blog *Wait but Why* (the link is listed in the Resources section) to gain a true appreciation for the artistic possibilities of simple lines and circles. You grew up drawing, but at some point somebody told you it was a waste of time and you should stop. So you stopped, and now you think you can't draw, but you can. All you need is the encouragement of friends and a willingness to accept failure and keep drawing.

It wasn't so long ago, in the age before cameras, printers, and copiers, that drawing was taught in school along with math, history, and science. Drawings were needed in order to convey information visually. It was a critical skill, especially in college biology, where freshmen took daily drawing courses. Why? Because it forced them to learn how to observe. But the benefits of drawing go far beyond honing our ability to look closely at the world. It encourages us to see everyday objects, even soup cans, in a new way that elevates them beyond the ordinary. Drawing is often used as therapy because it encourages us to be in the present moment, to quiet the mind and ease stress, much like with meditation. As humans, we feel intrinsically drawn to the pleasure of creating something out of nothing.

Are you ready to give drawing another try? If so, gather together with sketch pads, pencils, and erasers (dollar store materials are great for beginners) and Draw on This.

Let go of your desire for perfection—this is, after all, a sketching tutorial for beginners—then:

1 Select any object in the room that you want to draw. You don't all have to choose the same object. It's better if you don't so that you reduce the likelihood of artistic jealousy.

2 Loosely sketch the object you've selected. Don't grip your pencil so tightly that it leaves little indentations in your finger and thumb. You want to stay relaxed throughout the exercise.

3 Once you've completed an initial loose sketch, look for areas in the composition that need improvement and lightly pencil over them until you get closer to your desired result.

4 Keep going. Refine what you've sketched until you get even closer to the look you're striving for.

5 Now you're ready to use more confident lines to define the shape of your sketch. You can erase the scribbly lines from earlier steps, or let them disappear naturally under your bold contours.

Finally, it's time for a friendly show-and-tell where you display your work in a sketchy exhibition (if you're feeling particularly artistic, feel free to title your drawing). Can you match the sketch with the artist? What did you experience? Was there even the tiniest exhilaration in producing something you didn't think you were capable of? If so, keep drawing. If you have a family member who's an artist, you may want to do as Julie did and share your drawing with them along with a note saying, "Look what I did. Told you I could draw!" There are countless online drawing tutorials on YouTube: search for "beginner drawing lessons." We also recommend two books by Mark Kistler: *You Can Draw in 30 Days* or, if that seems like too long to achieve artistry, *You Can Draw It in Just 30 Minutes*.

Draw on This will help the most adamant left-brainer of your friends to believe in her creativity. Isn't that what friends are for? To make us believers in ourselves and draw out our potential?

26

A Friendly Time Capsule

MAKE A FUTURE ARCHAEOLOGIST TRY TO FIGURE OUT THE PURPOSE OF A THONG

"Prisoners, instead of being conveyed to the
several police stations in automobile patrol
wagons, will be sent through pneumatic tubes."
THE DETROIT CENTURY BOX FROM 1900

PREDICTS ELON MUSK'S HYPERLOOP

THE INTERNATIONAL TIME Capsule Society estimates that
there are between 10,000 and 15,000 time capsules world-
wide, encapsulating our collective yearning to speak to the
future. The earliest time capsule we know about was dated
from 1777 and discovered in 2017 in Burgos, Spain. It was
a wooden statue of Jesus that contained a document of economic, cultural, and political information—the Twitter feed of
the day—written by chaplain Joaquín Mínguez.

The world's most famous time capsule, the Westinghouse
Time Capsule, is a bullet-shaped copper tube that includes
messages from Thomas Mann and Albert Einstein, along with

carefully selected items to communicate with people five thousand years in the future. It was buried in 1938 at the precise moment of the autumnal equinox, on the eve of World War II and in the depths of an economic depression. The capsule weighs 800 pounds and is located fifty feet below the site of the 1939 New York World's Fair, in Flushing Meadows Park. The location is marked with a stone that hopefully nobody, including Mother Nature, will move for the next few thousand years.

The Westinghouse capsule contains a spool of thread, a fountain pen, an alphabet block set, and seventy-five types of fabrics, metals, plastics, and seeds. It also includes modern literature, contemporary art, Camel cigarettes, copies of *Life* magazine, and a Mickey Mouse watch. Ten million words on microfilm chronicling the events of the early twentieth century make up the news portion of the time capsule. Its creators anticipated that in five thousand years technology would progress beyond microfilm; therefore the capsule includes instructions for how to make both a microfilm viewer and a newsreel projector.

The items in the Westinghouse capsule were intended to reflect twentieth-century life in the United States. Both Thomas Mann and Albert Einstein wrote messages to the future, but with the world on the verge of war and economic uncertainty, neither seemed overly optimistic about the fate of humanity. Albert Einstein noted that "our time is rich in inventive minds," and "anyone who thinks about the future must live in fear and terror." Mann noted, "We know now that the idea of the future as a 'better world' was a fallacy of the doctrine of progress." Yikes! We hope that five thousand years from now, some academic from a more enlightened society will say the twentieth century was populated by pessimistic people.

Despite the doom and gloom of two great men, the New York World's Fair that featured the famous time capsule stressed optimism at its exhibits, and the soulful belief that one cannot address the future without fully understanding the present.

It is with this optimistic spirit that we challenge you to create A Friendly Time Capsule. This is your opportunity to collect artifacts that intentionally reflect your perspective of the present and will communicate with future versions of yourselves. Don't worry about how you'll manage to dig a hole fifty feet deep or make a copper capsule that can withstand five thousand years of corrosion. The idea behind A Friendly Time Capsule is to commemorate your friendship symbolically and send meaningful messages into your future.

Choose a container that somehow symbolizes your relationship and contents that speak to each of you individually and collectively, as friends, and the journey you've taken together. A handbag, beach bag, or decorative tin might be the most appropriate vehicle for transporting your collection of friendly treasures into the future. To generate ideas for the time capsule's contents, consider what you mean to each other and what you've done together. Books that you've shared, photographs of your get-togethers, and souvenirs collected on your travels with one another are a few suggestions.

For us, the most intriguing artifacts may prove to be the letters that we wrote to each other and to ourselves. The best way to make the future happen is to visualize it, and writing it down in the form of a letter to yourself can strengthen that vision. Maybe you'll want to describe where you see yourself in five or ten years from now, or perhaps you'll simply want to remind yourself of something you might not otherwise remember about this time in your life. Letters to each other can be expressions of gratitude, descriptions of particularly meaningful events you've shared, or even your predictions for the future.

In addition to letters, we each added three artifacts of historical importance, one of which was a thong that Deb placed in our time capsule to test two hypotheses: would it still fit her in 2020, and would a thong still be her preferred style of panty?

Taking the lead from Westinghouse, deposit your time capsule in its hiding place on a date and time that is special to you. Spring solstice is often associated with fertile rituals that are profoundly womanly, or perhaps you have a meaningful anniversary or want to mark the occasion of sealing your time capsule on a relevant date from your friend calendar. When we prepared our capsule in 2012, we decided to keep it covered for eight years. The first year of a new decade, 2020, is here, and we look forward to traveling back in time when we retrieve the messages from our past selves from the Lululemon bag in Julie's closet.

When you celebrate sealing your time capsule, set the date for an even more celebratory unsealing in the future, mark it in your calendars, and be sure to note where you put it!

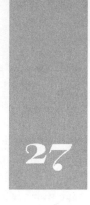

Ages Eight and Up
IT'S GOT TO BE EASY, RIGHT???

"Every child is an artist. The problem is
how to remain an artist once we grow up."
PABLO PICASSO

WHEN RESEARCHERS AT MIT wanted to test how rapid-transit systems could affect the city of Boston, they created a model using LEGO. LEGO? Yes, LEGO. MIT has used LEGO in several studies, proving that children's toys aren't necessarily child's play. Children reap the benefits of spatial, geometric, and architectural thinking, which are strengthened in constructive play and predictive of success in later life. But no child has ever said, "I'm developing my spatial awareness" when building with LEGO. She's having fun.

In his book *Wonderland*, Steven Johnson traces the origins of programmable machines to ancient music boxes and asserts that many new ideas came into the world simply because they're fun. When did we stop having fun playing with arts and crafts that came in a box, with a minimum age requirement like ages eight and up? There is no maximum age for this act of friendship, so go to a crafty store and find a kit that appeals to your inner child. If you're fearless, select matryoshka (Russian nesting doll) painting, glitter art, or a make-your-own volcano. Origami, crochet art, and balloon modeling are better choices for friends who want to keep their host's playroom free of glitter, or explosions, or (ye gods!) glitter explosions. Glitter has been aptly called the herpes of craft supplies, because once you have it, it's impossible to get rid of it.

Your inner child will have a ball with Ages Eight and Up, but that's not all: when your hands and mind are immersed in papier-mâché, a clay pot, or a pile of LEGO bricks, they're connected to the physical world and at a safe distance from the digital world where—face it—many of us spend far too much time. Ages Eight and Up is an ideal remedy for a particular set of modern anxieties—too much work, too much news, too much Internet. And who knows, as you're playing, your mind may wander to the solution of a vexing problem or a new idea. Girolamo Cardano was an Italian polymath who played with dice and discovered probability theory, a transformative idea that created job opportunities for epidemiologists, actuaries, and game theorists.

Complete the art or craft according to the instructions on your kit (or wing it) while your friends do likewise, and then compare your results and share any key discoveries. Be sure to present a prize to the woman whose work most closely resembles the pictured finished product that came with her kit. A failed attempt at creating a velvet Elvis or kinetic sand art make terrific prizes.

We don't *always* recommend wine as an accompaniment to acts of friendship, but it may be a good pairing with Ages Eight and Up, particularly if papier-mâché and balloons are involved and you want to create something truly original and scary. And remember: friends don't let friends glitter!

28

Standing Jokes

"HAVE YOU HEARD ABOUT THE RESTAURANT ON THE MOON? GREAT FOOD, BUT NO ATMOSPHERE."

"The worst time to have a heart attack is during a game of charades."
DEMETRI MARTIN

ON THE EVE of his ninety-fifth birthday, comedian Bob Hope told *TV Guide* that the secret to his longevity wasn't diet and exercise. "Laughter is it," he said, adding, "Laughter is therapy—an instant vacation." Often when friends get together an instant vacation of laughter is the result, so a friendly gathering is the perfect environment in which to consciously tickle your funny bones and massage your souls. As we mentioned in Mock Therapy (Act 10), laughing burns calories, lowers blood pressure, and reduces stress. It also increases immune response while you work your abdominal, respiratory, and facial muscles. Michael Miller of the University of Maryland Medical Center and author of a study on the effects of laughter on endothelial cells—they like it!—longs for the day when doctors all over the world start recommending that everyone laugh for at least fifteen to twenty minutes every day in the same way they recommend a minimum thirty minutes of exercise.

One of the first government actions in Nazi Germany was the establishment of a law that made anti-Nazi humor an act of treason. Humor is one of the most effective antidotes for brainwashing, and the most enjoyable form of self-medication. With humor, an overwhelming situation can feel manageable, and the brain—freed from the debilitating inertia of stress—can think of creative solutions.

When was the last time you told a joke? Sharing jokes through social media is commonplace, but there aren't too many people who take the social risk of telling a joke in person. Nonetheless, having an inventory of jokes can come in handy at a cocktail party, a family gathering, or even a job interview. "Can you tell me a joke?" is a great but terrifying interview question. You can tell a lot about a person by the joke they choose and how they tell it, while not having a joke to tell is also revealing.

Standing Jokes will give you an opportunity to test your comedic material on your friends so that you can draw a rapt audience at your next family birthday dinner and won't be caught humorless at your next job interview. Telling jokes is a skill that draws on many talents—acting, memorization, timing, and confidence—and it can be learned. The most important element of success is committing yourself one hundred percent to the joke. If you're not sure your joke is good, this uncertainty will come across in the delivery and it won't be funny.

For Standing Jokes, select three jokes that made you laugh the first time you heard them. They can be mild, medium, and hot: jokes for job interviews; jokes for friends and family; or jokes for after-midnight at cocktail parties. Rehearse your routine several times until you have comfortably memorized it and can perform it smoothly while maintaining eye contact with your audience, rather than looking up at the ceiling trying to remember exactly what the octopus said to the turtle. Or was it the other way around? No, it wasn't a turtle, it was a frog. Or a pollywog. Yes. A pollywog wiggled up to a bar...

On the evening of the activity, create a comedy club atmosphere (minus the hecklers) with a darkened room and a stage with a tall wooden stool and a glass of water. If you're daring, make Standing Jokes into a comedic competition, where the friend who tells the joke that cracks everyone up the most wins a Standing Joke "trophy" (rubber chicken, whoopee cushion, fake doo-doo—the possibilities are endless).

If you want the laughs but not the challenge of Standing Jokes, queue up your favorite stand-up comedian on Netflix or YouTube. (We have included a few recommendations in the Resources section.) If you want to ramp up the challenge and turn Standing Jokes into an adventure, make up your own jokes.

To help you develop your comedy routine, use the Jerry Seinfeld "Pop-Tart" method. First, be open to noticing what you think is funny, no matter how small or insignificant it may seem. For example, "Pop-Tart" is a fun and insignificant thing to say. This is your starting point. Seinfeld wants the first line to be funny right away, so he says, "When I was a kid and they invented the Pop-Tart, the back of my head blew right off." Notice how it was a specific part of Seinfeld's head that blew off, not the whole thing. This little detail makes the line funnier. And of course he's lying: the back of Seinfeld's head didn't blow off, or he wouldn't be well enough to tell the joke. It's okay to lie when you tell a joke. In fact, it's good to tell a jokey lie.

Then Seinfeld adds context to explain *why* the back of his head blew off. It was the 1960s and breakfast consisted of toast, wood-chipper Shredded Wheat, and years-old frozen orange juice. It was into this barren breakfast landscape that the Pop-Tart popped. The way Seinfeld describes it, kids were like chimps playing in the dirt with sticks when the alien spacecraft *Pop-Tart* appeared. Chimps, dirt, playing, and sticks. Seinfeld uses as many funny words as he can cram into a sentence and he makes sure that the funniest bit always comes at the end of the joke. The beautiful Pop-Tart world that Kellogg created in the 1960s felt so perfect—two slots in the toaster, two Pop-Tarts—with the same shape (and nutritional content) as their packaging. One wouldn't be enough and three are too many, but Seinfeld realizes there never was a problem with the number of Pop-Tarts in a package: "They can't go stale because they were never fresh." *Da-dum*!

Your turn. It doesn't take many attempts at joke-making to gain an appreciation for the talent (and stamina) of comics who can take the stage and be funny for ninety minutes.

We hope that you enjoy this act of friendship so much that it becomes an agenda item whenever you get together, and the Standing Joke trophy for the funniest friend becomes...um... a standing joke.

29

May I Have a Word?

IS A "SNICKERSNEE" A GIGGLE, A MINIATURE CHOCOLATE BAR, OR A KNIFE?

"I like the word 'indolence.' It makes my laziness seem classy."

BERN WILLIAMS

YOUR BRAIN LOVES wordplay. More specifically, your Broca's area loves wordplay. The Broca is the area of the brain involved in language processing and is named after the person who identified it, French physician Paul Broca. You can thank your Broca's area for your ability to consume the 100,000 words the University of California estimates that you see in a single day. Most of the time you'll skip right over them, not paying attention, until you hit an unfamiliar word that gives you a little jolt of surprise, or one used playfully that delivers a hit of dopamine when you catch the double meaning of a pun.

A person who gets textual pleasure from words and wordplay is called a lexophile. Etymology tells us where a word comes from, when it was first heard, and how it has changed over time. The etymology of the word "etymology" combines *etymos*, meaning "true" and *logia*, meaning "study." Therefore etymology is the study of the true meaning of words.

New words are added to the dictionary every year because they have been used often and consistently. Among the list of a thousand new words (and old words with new meanings) that were added to the *Merriam-Webster Dictionary* in 2019 are: screen time (time spent in front of a screen that used to mean the time actors appeared onscreen in a movie); go-cup (a plastic or paper cup used especially for taking a beverage off the premises of a bar, restaurant, and so on); garbage time (the final moments of a game when one side has an insurmountable lead); unplug (refrain from using electronic devices); and buzzy (characterized by a lot of excited talk or attention). *The game was buzzy, but once her screen time turned into garbage time she grabbed a go-cup and unplugged . . .*

Words are a bit like people in that they have a personality. Words can be fun, complicated, sexy, or offensive. We often react to words emotionally and judgmentally. For example, many people don't like the word "moist." There's even a Facebook group with nearly 3,000 likes that is called "I HATE the word MOIST," and Jimmy Fallon sarcastically thanked moist for being the worst word ever. As reported on *Mental Floss*, researchers from Oberlin College in Ohio and Trinity University in San Antonio ran three experiments to gauge how many people dislike the word moist and why. It turned out that more than twenty percent of the population studied had an aversion to the word, but not because of the way it sounds. The association of moist with bodily functions is what seems to turn people off.

The meanings (personalities) of a word can change over time, too. Consider that the word "wench" (Old English origin from the word *wenchel,* meaning children of either sex) evolved to mean "female child" and later came to be used to refer to women servants—and more pejoratively to "wanton women." And the word "awful" used to mean "worthy of awe," which is how we got expressions like "the awful majesty of God." Speaking of "worthy of awe" we now have the all-too-familiar word that has lost its way and drifted into the mundane: awesome.

Even our names have origins and meaning, and research suggests that they are a kind of a self-fulfilling prophesy: we tend to look and act the part of our names. Roses tend to act feminine and Graces tend to exude grace. Deb found out that the name "Deborah" is from the Hebrew word meaning "bee," and if you ask her two younger sisters, they'd probably tell you that it should be "Queen Bee." As for Julie, her name has English and French origins and means "youthful." That makes sense to us, as her family's roots are in England, and Julie has a love for all things French. Lynne's real first name is Sandra, a derivative of Cassandra from Greek mythology whose punishment for her deception of Apollo was to make predictions nobody believed. When she worked as a pharmaceutical forecaster, nobody believed Lynne/Sandra's predictions. Name etymologies are positively spooky!

The activity May I Have a Word? puts the spotlight on the words we say—funny, new, odd, and misquoted words. It's an activity that challenges you to expand your vocabulary, explore the fascinating origins of common words, and tell stories about word blunders.

Before your next get-together, choose a word you've recently encountered ("shambolic" for example). At your gathering, share your word and where you found it ("[Magic Johnson] left in his wake a shambolic franchise," from a *Washington Post* article by Cindy Boren), along with its etymology (from "shambles," meaning disorder). Tell everyone your favorite word (for example, Julie loves the word "wiener" because it's funny to say); least favorite word (Deb's one of the twenty-plus percent who doesn't like the word "moist"); a word you might have heard but, in print, looks different than you expected (Deb expected "albeit" to be three words, *all be it*); and a word or phrase you have misused (for example, "grilled cheese"... as a child Lynne thought it was "girl cheese"). Keep the etymology going and share the origin of your name. When was it first used? Any particular reason why your parents gave you that name? Do you feel like your name suits you, or would you choose another one?

According to a study by Marc Brysbaert and others from Ghent University in Belgium, the average native English-speaking American will know around 42,000 words by the time they are twenty years old, but will only learn 6,000 additional words in the next forty years. Considering this, May I Have a Word? is a fun way to increase your vocabulary beyond 48,000 words by age sixty.

Oh, and by the way, besides being fun to say out loud, a "snickersnee" is a large knife that began its life as a word when two Dutch words, *steken* (to thrust) and *snijden* (to cut) mated. Etymology can be so sexy!

30

Collage Life

COMBINE THE MIXED
ELEMENTS THAT ARE YOU

"Life is like a collage. Its individual pieces are arranged
to create harmony. Appreciate the artwork of your life."
AMY LEIGH MERCREE

YOU MAY THINK that collage is for kids with scissors, glue sticks,
and magazines, but you've likely never seen Jason Mecier's
portraits of Amy Winehouse made out of pills, of Joan Riv-
ers constructed out of beauty products, or of Hugh Hefner
made out of *Playboy* magazines. Collage has a clever way of
adding a subtext that makes the familiar look unfamiliar, or
even unsettling.

Art history books often credit Picasso with inventing collage
around 1912, and making it a distinctive feature of modern
art, but this is once again the case of a man taking credit for
women's work. Collage (from the French word *coller*, meaning
"glue") dates back at least sixty years *before* Picasso to Victorian
era where women used a cut-and-paste technique combining

photographs and watercolors, and displayed their work—some that wouldn't look out of place as examples of Modernist art—in the anonymous art galleries that were their homes. Collage Life is a celebration of these overlooked women artists who practiced the collage technique and used it for witty or mischievous ends—for example, featuring people suspended in a spider's web, mimicking the entanglements of high society—long before a man gave it artistic credibility.

The best collages put art and life together in unexpected ways that make us pause and think. In her book *Collage, Assemblage, and the Found Object,* Diane Waldman writes that collage brings "the incongruous in meaningful congress with the ordinary." In other words, collage is the perfect medium for making a visual representation of the fantastical elements that compose you. When you do the activity Collage Life, think of your art as the surrealists did—a way to reveal your true subconscious essence—or simply have fun with your friends as you stick random stuff that "speaks to you" on a piece of poster board. It's a good idea to scan the Internet for examples of collage to put yourself in the Alice-in-Wonderland mindset that makes this form of art so whimsical.

Before you take scissors to magazines, photos of yourself, or (like collage artist Kurt Schwitters) anything found on the streets of Berlin, take a moment to reflect on who you are. Close your eyes, take a deep breath, and think back to when you were a child. Use your journal to jot down a few key words as you contemplate your essence.

What were you like then? What did you enjoy doing? What did you do on your summer vacations? What role did you play in your family?

Now think about a young adult version of you. Where did you spend your time? What were your interests?

Finally, who are you today? What do you do with your time? What are your values? Is it a picture of Rosa Parks or Lady Gaga that resonates most with you? Does skiing, running, or skydiving strike a chord?

Once your mind is a mix of past, present, and aspirational versions of yourself, select your source material. Magazines and Internet images are the easiest to cut and paste, but there's nothing stopping you from making a collage out of found objects such as shells, snippets from books, or old family photos. If you choose to go the magazine or Internet route, look for words, photographs, or illustrations that you find appealing, and try not to curb your impulses.

Once everyone has collaged to exhaustion, it's time for show-and-tell. As a prelude to the formal presentation, you may wish to have an exhibition where you display your unsigned masterpieces and play match the friend to the collage. Did your friends correctly match your collage to you? If not, why? Is something missing? Is something illustrated that doesn't seem to fit with who you are? When you present your collage to the group, ask your friends what they see, rather than explaining how it expresses who you are. Is there any gap between your self-rendition and how you present yourself to others? Another spin on this activity is to have a Collage Life marathon, where you make collages of yourselves *and* each other.

Collages make great keepsakes. Take yours out from time to time and compare what you're doing now with how you saw yourself when you created your masterpiece. Julie keeps her collage at the bottom of her night table, preserved under books, and Deb has hers folded in a shoebox in her closet. Lynne's collage is in an indeterminate place, where it's residing with the countless other treasures she threw away on a minimalist binge but shouldn't have. A collage, even one that has disappeared, can be a reminder of the random items of which we're made.

The disparity between real life and Collage Life may prompt you to make changes or to resurrect a long-forgotten project. Before you roll up your masterpiece, look for playful messages

from your unconscious mind that you can cut and paste onto
your real life, evidence that you have channeled the mischievous spirit of the Victorian women artists who brought collage
to life.

31

A Night at the Improv

YOU JUST LANDED ON
A DESERTED ISLAND. GO!

"The rules of improvisation apply beautifully to life.
Never say no, you have to be interested to be interesting, and your job is to support your partners."

SCOTT ADSIT

HAVE YOU EVER wanted to silence your inner critic, the
voice inside your head that always says, "No!" when "Hell,
yes!" is what you want to say? Technically speaking, improvisation is a form of acting and reacting from the imagination,
without a script or premeditative thought, but what improv is
truly about is *letting go*. Jazz musicians, freestyle rappers, and
improv comedians talk about stepping into an alternative
reality beyond time, where the mind is free of thoughts and
everything seems to flow. The state of flow is what psychologist
Mihaly Csikszentmihalyi (no, that's not an improvised name)
famously associated, not with happiness, but with happiness's
more spiritual cousin: contentment.

As reported in the *Washington Post*, neuroscientists have scanned the brains of rappers during a freestyle session and compared them with brains reciting memorized raps. What they found was astounding: rappers who improvise bypass many of the brain's conscious control centers to tap into a well of pure inspiration. Studies of jazz musicians had similar findings: the thought process of improvisation gives musicians access to patterns and combinations of sounds that the inhibited mind, the part of us bound by the familiar and acceptable, can't access. It may seem like an option to increase the level of difficulty of artistic performance, but some scientists believe that improvisation has been crucial to our species' survival and a fundamental part of what it means to be human. If we responded without the ability to improvise, reacting in a limited number of ways to everything that happened to us, not only would life be a robotic bore, but we wouldn't last long in an ever-changing world.

You may not be able to freestyle like Snoop Dogg or play improv piano like Thelonious Monk, but you can hone your improvisational skills by pretending you're an improv comedian co-starring with your friends in A Night at the Improv.

The key to successful improv is to go with the flow, to build on your partner's ideas, no matter how outlandish they may be. When you accept the ridiculous without hesitation or judgment, together with your friends you can explore new, wildly creative worlds. And who doesn't want to explore wild new worlds with their friends?

The skill that is essential for improv is the same skill that is essential to be a great conversationalist. Listening. While your partner is performing, you shouldn't try to think of something funny or plan what you're going to say: you should pay close attention. Introverts accustomed to pondering their replies will find improv challenging, but (like Think on Your Stilettos, Act 16) it's good for them. You're not looking for perfection in improv. You're looking for "yes" instead of "no," and to welcome the unexpected.

Improv forces you to stay in the moment, to connect with the absurd theater of your subconscious, and to follow and support the efforts of others. It's a superb mental and physical exercise that challenges you to be creative in mind and body, and improv is a great metaphor for life. If you can take whatever improv (or life) throws at you and play with it creatively, you will thrive. Every time you respond to what's happening with "yes, and..." rather than "no, but..." you move the story of your life forward.

You might find A Night at the Improv intimidating. You may think that you have to be a manic comedian like Robin Williams was, or that you need special acting skills to participate, but the truth is that improv is a skill of subtraction, of letting go of your inhibitions. The goal of improv is to react through words and actions to an imaginary situation. The key to success is to *fully believe* in the world you create with your imagination. We are all born perfect improvisers; it's only as we get older that we begin to follow a script.

Letting go of your script, even for A Night at the Improv, is an invaluable exercise because it's a live demonstration of how your personality is nothing but a collection of habitual actions. Change your actions and reactions, and suddenly you become a different person.

Are you ready to use the magic of improvisation to become a different person? Gather for some group improv, select two people to go first, and have one person draw a scenario from a hat.

You can dream up your own prompts or use our favorite scenarios/opening lines listed here:

· A late-night Uber...

· Two spies run into each other at the supermarket...

- The first women to land on Mars ...

- A superhero enters a bar ...

- The world's worst hairdresser ...

- A dentist discovers something unusual ...

- An underwear model goes rogue ...

- Two criminals are on the run ...

- Two strangers are trapped in an elevator ...

- A first date where neither person resembles the dating website photo ...

- A bride refuses to go down the aisle ...

- A talk show host interviews an unusual guest ...

- A flight attendant makes an unexpected announcement ...

- An audition for a commercial ...

- An alien from another planet has arrived at the door ...

- A woman is hiring a private detective ...

- "There's something I have to tell you ..."

- "Don't touch that!"

- "Didn't you see the sign?"

- "I'm so excited to meet you!!! May I have your autograph?"

- "Do you remember how I got this tattoo?"

- "I'd like to return this sex toy ..."

Okay, we'll stop now.

Set a timer for sixty seconds or however long you'd like to play out the scenario, and when the time is up, switch to a fresh pair of improvisers and scene. Or someone from the audience can call out "Freeze!" and take over from the point where the scene was frozen, replacing the actor for whichever character she'd like to play.

Remember that the secret to improv is "Yes, and . . ." It's all about accepting what someone has to offer and building on it. Relax, connect with your body, and let go of your inhibitions. Think of A Night at the Improv as a way to loosen the grip of personality and mute your inner critic. We encourage you to use it as an excuse to try on some dramatically different personas among the supportive "Yes, ands . . ." of friends.

32

Close-Knit Friends

HAVE EVERYONE IN STITCHES!

"Properly practiced, knitting soothes the troubled
spirit, and it doesn't hurt the untroubled spirit either."
ELIZABETH ZIMMERMAN

AS PEOPLE SEARCH for ways to unwind, relax, and disconnect from the digital world, the craft of knitting is enjoying a
renaissance, but you may be surprised to learn that knitting is
an activity that has been traced back to socks from the elev-
enth century. Discovered in Egypt, these cozy artifacts appear
to have been worn by a two-toed human, making them both
the world's first knitted item *and* the world's first toe socks! It's
believed that knitting began in the Middle East and came to
Europe via trade routes where it became so popular that even
the Virgin Mary was depicted as a knitter in paintings such as
Knitting Madonna by Bertram of Minden. The fact that there
were no ancient legends about knitting (although there were
legendary spinners and weavers) makes historians believe that
knitting is a relatively recent invention that's older than cro-
cheting and younger than weaving.

Although today we think of knitting as a mostly feminine pastime, during the Middle Ages the occupation was exclusively male and strictly controlled by guilds. It took six years of training to become a Master Knitter—three years of apprenticeship and three years of traveling the medieval world in search of new patterns and techniques—that culminated in a practical exam. Each candidate for Master Knitter had thirteen weeks to create a series of pieces such as a cap, shirt, or gloves, and the ultimate expression of skill, a knitted carpet displaying intricate patterns in multiple colors of wool.

Within the hypermasculine history of knitting there are military yarns. During the Crimean War, James Thomas Brudenell wore a knitted vest into battle. The style became fashionable and was named after Brudenell's aristocratic title: the Seventh Earl of *Cardigan*. During the First World War, knitting was considered a patriotic duty, and the Red Cross mobilized knitters across the United States to fulfill a request for over 1.5 million garments. Wounded soldiers joined the effort from their hospital beds and knitted to mentally and physically occupy themselves as they recovered.

Today, many knitters use their needles as a form of self-care that is both meditative *and* productive. According to Carrie Barron, a psychiatrist, director of creativity for resilience at Dell Medical School, and co-author of *The Creativity Cure*, knitting can lower blood pressure and improve mental health. Knitting has even been shown to reduce awareness of chronic pain.

In the beginning, you'll need to focus on the task at hand, but once your hands settle into the knitting rhythm, your brain can drift away comfortably into a state of relaxation that Chris Bailey, an avid knitter and the author of *Hyperfocus,* calls "scatterfocus." The rhythmic, meditative nature of knitting engages the mind in a healthy way that keeps stressful thoughts away, yet encourages gentle reflection and creative insights. And while your hands are on your needles, they're off your smartphone, making knitting an ideal activity to lure you away from the vortex of the digital world.

When asked to describe their mood *before* knitting, thirty-four percent of knitters surveyed in a study published in the *British Journal of Occupational Therapy* reported feeling "happy" and twenty-three percent reported being "a little sad" to "very sad." When asked to report their mood post-knitting, less than one percent remained sad and eighty-one percent described themselves as "a little happy" to "very happy."

Perhaps the reason knitting makes us happy is because it satisfies both sides of the brain. Learning new patterns—some can be complicated—occupies the left side of your brain and improves motor skills and cognitive memory, while the right hemisphere gets to play, creatively and artistically. And knitting is productive: the fruits of your labor are useful items that keep us comfy and cozy—and we all know how satisfying it is to give handmade gifts.

For many folks, once they learn to knit, they can't stop. There are always new patterns, different types of yarn, and various techniques to try out. When their families and friends have all the knitted garments they can handle, many yarn crafters continue to knit and purl for charity... or as a form of protest. "I never associated knitting with having as much power as my science, and now I'm realizing that it really does," said Heidi Arjes, a postdoctoral fellow at Stanford and designer of the "resistor" knit cap. Her beanies feature a battery, three resistors, and a closed circuit pattern to celebrate women in science, technology, engineering, and math for the March for Science. Schooled in science and skilled in art, Heidi says, "Knitting is a way I can reach people."

Are you ready to reach out to your friends and knit your way to happy? If there is already a knitter in your group, invite her to share her knowledge as described in Live and Let's Learn (Act 45). When we did Close-Knit Friends, Lynne surprised herself and all present by remembering a decades-old knitting skill, which she tried to teach Deb, whose needles were small and slippery, adding to the degree of difficulty. To prepare for this activity, Lynne had been to a knitting shop where she found Jenny, who sat knitting in a chair. Jenny told Lynne which needles to buy, spun her yarn, and warned her not to drink wine and knit.

If there isn't an expert like Jenny in your group to keep you in stitches, there are countless beginner knitter tutorials available online—in the Resources section you can find the link to a popular introductory video to help you get started. Beginners could also use large diameter yarn, purchase a knitting kit to create a specific project, or try out the Close-Knit Friends activity to make a scarf, the quintessential beginner item. But here's a twist: plan a knitting circle and task everyone to create a length of the scarf that the lucky recipient—the knitter whose work everyone agrees is most impressive—will stitch together into a single piece. After you've completed your first project you'll be hooked and ready to try your hand at something else. A baby blanket? A doggie mat? A wine-bottle cozy? Before you know it, you'll be ready to knit a carpet and earn your Master Knitter status.

So cast off and let the stress unravel as you become Close-Knit Friends.

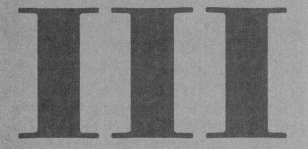

III

acts of adventure

"As soon as I saw you, I knew an adventure was about to happen."

WINNIE THE POOH

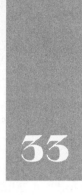

33

And Now for Something *Completely* Different

GIVE YOUR BRAIN A DOSE OF VITAMIN *NEW*

"Serve the dinner backward, do anything—
but for goodness' sake, do something weird."
ELSA MAXWELL

IMAGINE A WORLD in which you never got bored. Netflix, video games, and our boredom-busting smartphones would lose significant appeal. You'd never have to deal with that depressing "the thrill is gone" feeling, but you'd also never feel the spark of creativity that nudges you out of boredom and into new experiences.

There's a fancy term for why we get bored. When we adapt to what's new and return to a stable level of contentment, we're on what's called a "hedonic treadmill." We habitually jump on the boring hedonic treadmill because if we didn't adapt, everything would seem new all the time. Imagine your new car never losing its appeal. Also imagine never being able to get over that awful breakup. From an evolutionary perspective, we need the boredom of the hedonic treadmill for survival: if we never registered something completely different as a potential new reward or threat, we could easily miss what could help or harm us.

David Foster Wallace describes how the hedonic treadmill works in "Shipping Out," a story about his week-long experience on a luxury cruise ship. At first he orders room service and feels he must justify his indulgence to the cabin steward who delivers it by scattering pretend work on his bed. But by the end of the cruise he's dialing up his meal and becoming angrily impatient when his food hasn't arrived in fifteen minutes! Another common example of the hedonic treadmill involves winning the lottery. Lottery winners feel a flush of joy when they win and will often surround themselves with luxury items, but soon these treasures become commonplace, and winners are no happier than they were before they hit the jackpot.

So the good *and* bad news is that your brain can adjust to any environment of extreme gratification—or major disappointment—and has an insatiable craving for novelty. Have you ever driven along a familiar route and zoned out to the point where you couldn't remember most of your journey? Compare that experience with one of driving through a city you've never visited before, and a neighborhood that doesn't appear to be particularly friendly. Your brain switches on and becomes much more attentive when you feed it something different. It's that aliveness that we want to tap into with the acts of friendship in this book, which offers dozens of ways to break from routine, expand your horizons, and wake up your brain, specifically the substantia nigra/ventral tegmental area—let's call it the novelty center—which plays a large role in learning and memory. In an "oddball experiment," where subjects were exposed to familiar, less familiar, and completely new things, only the completely new things tickled the novelty center and increased activity in the dopamine pathways where reward chemicals are dispensed.

Have you ever wondered why you can remember details from your teens and twenties in high definition, but trying to remember what you did last weekend feels like grasping for the answer to a tough trivia question? This phenomenon, based on a study of thousands of autobiographical recollections, has been called the "reminiscence bump." The theory behind the reminiscence bump suggests that the reason our memories of adolescence and early adulthood are so clear is because that was when we were experiencing many life changes for the first time.

And Now for Something *Completely* Different encourages you to reactivate the reminiscence bump by doing things for the first time. Finding quirky ways to interact with your friends will enable you to jump off the hedonic treadmill, give your brain a dose of vitamin *New*, and create lasting memories. This activity involves gathering together to do three things you've never done before. Don't fret: you don't have to do anything that involves a bungee cord.

If you're drawing a blank, here's a list of completely different suggestions for inspiration:

- Dressing up in evening wear, pajamas, or a costume for no reason at all
- Having breakfast for dinner
- Using all glassware to serve your meal
- Listening to a type of music you don't usually listen to
- Inviting someone new into your social circle
- Sitting on the floor instead of on the sofa or a chair
- Eating with your hands

Having a "girls' night in" where you dress up in evening gowns to eat macaroni and cheese with chopsticks while listening to death metal is guaranteed to perk up your brain ... along with the brain of anyone else who finds out what you're up to. We'll never forget the night we sat on the floor in our pajamas and high heels eating quiche from crystal coffee mugs while listening to the Delta blues.

Here's to creating some *completely* different memories.

34

Move Ya Body

PASS AROUND *THIS*
MIRACLE DRUG

"Exercising is better than any drug or anything
else we have for aging. There's no downside.
If this were a drug, it would be the safest,
most effective drug in the universe."
JAMES HILL

WE MOVE, THEREFORE we think. You've probably never
thought of movement as the reason you're able to put thoughts
together, but research confirms that we're born movers. It was
a mere ten thousand years ago, a New York minute on the evolutionary clock, that we were hunter-gatherers covering ten to
fourteen miles per day. That's 20,000 to 28,000 steps daily.
As we moved, our brains grew and we evolved. Now, the average person covers roughly 5,000 steps per day, a fraction of our
hunter-gatherer ancestors. If moving grew our brains, is a sedentary lifestyle shrinking them? Studies have shown that brain
mass increases with exercise, and without movement, our lives

shrink: a sedentary lifestyle is an incubator for depression, anxiety, and stress that kills IQ points and accelerates aging.

Have you ever wondered if your genes make you look old? Not if you engage in regular physical activity. Telomeres are the caps on the end of our DNA strands that protect our chromosomes, and are also markers of aging that will prematurely fray with excess stress. Physical activity can turn your telomeres into beautiful, long, willowy nucleotides, defying the effects of stress. The more you move forward, up, down, sideways, or in reverse, the more you turn the clock backward. And that's only the beginning. Exercise is first-line therapy for depression, burns off stress, and improves your sex life.

But wait, there's more!

Movement stimulates the release of norepinephrine, improving attention, perception, and motivation. Brain-derived neurotrophic factor (BDNF, also known as Miracle-Gro for the brain) is released when you exercise, protecting and repairing neurons—the nerve cells in the brain—from injury and degeneration. Hormones combine with BDNF to grow new brain cells, regulating mood and providing mental clarity. The hippocampus—the part of the brain associated with learning and memory—grows with exercise and becomes positively bodacious. Endorphins flow, dulling the sensation of pain, and serotonin is released, improving mood. Blood flow to the brain increases as the heart pounds harder and faster, delivering more oxygen and nutrients and improving waste disposal (believe us, you don't want waste accumulating in your brain). The feel-good hormone dopamine is released when we exercise, improving mood, focus, and learning.

And we haven't even talked about your left ventricle yet—how moving your body makes your heart stronger and more efficient, or how it boosts the capacity of mitochondria, the energy powerhouses in your muscles that, like telomeres, are markers of aging. Or how exercise leads to improved immune function, improved sleep, longer life... okay, we'll stop now, even though we could go on and on and on. Let's leave it at this: exercise is a little bit of Prozac, a little bit of Ritalin, and, thanks to endocannabinoids, a little bit of marijuana. If you want to read more about this miracle drug, we recommend John Ratey's *Spark*, Chris Crowley's *Younger Next Year*, and Elizabeth Blackburn and Elissa Epel's *The Telomere Effect*, for readers who enjoy mainlining the benefits of physical activity.

Exercise is undoubtedly a wonder drug, but the sweaty packaging and time commitment can be off-putting to some. Sweating with your friends, however, can be fun. If you do only one of our acts of friendship, please let it be Move Ya Body. Our bodies were meant to move. Together.

Never before in history have there been so many ways to move your body. If you want to turn physical activity into a true adventure, Move Ya Body in a *way* or a *place* that you never have before. For example, put on those hiking boots that you bought years ago, pack some water, bug spray, sun protection, and (unless you're familiar with edible plants) sustenance, and head to an unfamiliar hiking trail. Nature has an immediate de-stressing effect, so combining exercise, friendship, and the outdoors is one of the best things you can do for your mental and physical health.

If your idea of an adventure is dinner on a patio, consider a more urban workout you've never tried before—aerial yoga, Zumba, spinning, belly dancing (see Dances with Bellies, Act 21), disco kickboxing, or if you're particularly brave, a TRX suspension trainer class. Whatever Move Ya Body activity you choose, you will find your stamina increases, and the likelihood that you will get lost hiking in the wilderness decreases, when you're with friends.

One final enticement to get you moving with your friends that we couldn't resist: a study from researchers at Yale and Oxford published in *The Lancet* found that exercise is more important to your mental health than your economic status, and sociable exercise has the *most* positive effect on your well-being. So please plan a friend date to Move Ya Body!

35

Local Roots

DIG SOME REAL FOOD

"About eighty percent of the food on shelves of super-
markets today didn't exist a hundred years ago."
LARRY MCCLEARY

IT'S A FOOD minefield out there. From free-run, free-range,
cage-free, gluten-free, fat-free, omega-3, pasteurized, unpas-
teurized, grass-fed, grain-fed, farmed, farm-raised, wild to
GMO, non-GMO, organic—are there any foods that come
without adjective additives? How are you supposed to know
what to put into your shopping cart? You need a PhD in food
science to enter a grocery store if you want to interpret nutrition labels and figure out how to mix and match the items in
your cart.

It's not easy to be as cool as a cucumber with the latest grocery shopping rules: keep to the store perimeter, don't buy
anything with an ingredient you can't pronounce (food by
any chemical's name isn't food), avoid the dirty dozen (wasn't
that a '60s movie?), and steer the cart away from fake food (if

"cheese" isn't found in the refrigerated section, it isn't cheese). With all the talk about what we should and shouldn't eat coming from experts who aren't even in agreement, we're left not knowing what to buy, eat, or serve to our friends and families.

Prior to 1916 when the first grocery store to introduce self-service markets opened (called Piggly Wiggly, or as Deb calls it, "The Pig"), meals were prepared using seasonal fruits and vegetables, herbs from the garden, and livestock raised by a local farmer. Our ancestors may not have had the variety we have today, or the pleasure of eating blueberries in January, but they were eating *real* food with more taste, and they knew where it came from. Food grown within the U.S. travels an average of 1,500 miles to get to the grocery store—equivalent to the distance from Houston to Buffalo. And that banana that you ate for breakfast has likely come from Ecuador—in many cases, thousands of miles from plantation to table! The farther your "fresh" produce travels, the less nutritious (and tasty) it is by the time you eat it.

We challenge you to find Local Roots by foraging in your own community for something to eat. Get together with your friends at a local farmers' market or, better yet, a farm, and fill your baskets to the brim with foods that were nestled in the warmth of the earth's soil, or dangled from a branch bathed in sunshine, a few hours earlier. And if you're feeling adventurous, and if it's offered, take the opportunity to harvest the food yourself. Locally (and often organically) grown fruits and veggies will delight your senses, and may even trigger wonderful memories of grandma making jams and jellies in the kitchen.

Local Roots also feeds your mental health. A study published in the *Journal of Public Health* suggests that participating in local food projects may have a positive effect on wellbeing and psychological health. Lead researcher Zareen Bharucha said that "Community gardens, community supported agriculture, and farmers' markets, can bring people together, improve diets, improve connection to nature, and help people learn new things."

According to the U.S. Department of Agriculture, there were 8,687 farmers' markets operating in the United States in 2017, almost five times the number that there were in 1994. Search online to find a homegrown market close to you. Not only will you nourish your body with nature's best, but you and your friends may connect with other like-minded agritourists. Studies have shown that people who visit farmers' markets have ten times more conversations than they would at a supermarket. You might even speak directly with the farmer who worked tirelessly to plant and harvest the crops. Tickle your taste buds with samples of the fresh and/or unfamiliar produce plucked at their nutritional peak. What a delicious idea!

After you've filled your baskets full of fruits and vegetables of all colors of the rainbow, head back to a friend's home to make a beautiful salad with those fresh ingredients. Toss around your thoughts on your visit to the farmers' market, share some of your favorite food and drink discoveries—Deb is forever grateful to Julie for introducing her to locally-grown Riesling—and celebrate the bounty that began with Local Roots.

36

Testing the Waters

WHAT FLOATS YOUR BOAT?

"Where the waters do agree, it is
quite wonderful the relief they give."
JANE AUSTEN

WE ALL BEGAN life in amniotic fluid that consisted of ninety-eight percent water, and were born into bodies made up of about eighty percent water, declining to sixty percent by the time we reach adulthood. Perhaps because it's inherent to life itself, water draws so many of us to it and fills us with a sense of homecoming. Water seeps into every crack and crevice of life—we play in it, bathe in it, swim in it, wash most things in it, and drink it to survive. Clean water is essential to all of us and was recognized as a human right by the United Nations General Assembly in 2010.

Given how primal our relationship to water is, it should come as no surprise that being near water or in water douses us in happiness. One of the leading researchers on the health benefits of water is Wallace J. Nichols, marine biologist and author of *Blue Mind*. According to Nichols, the mere sight or sound of water promotes wellness by lowering the stress hormone cortisol, increasing the happy chemical serotonin, and inducing a state of calm. And drinking water lubricates the joints, keeps the digestive system flowing, maintains blood pressure, delivers oxygen throughout the body, and hydrates the skin. Even mild dehydration can impair brain function and make you cranky, tired, and anxious. Many factors contribute to how much water you should drink; the Mayo Clinic advises that your fluid intake is probably adequate if you rarely feel thirsty and your urine is colorless or light yellow.

Not to segue from urine to swimming, but with three-quarters of the earth's surface covered with water, it's only natural to plan a Testing the Waters activity, especially if you're lucky enough to live near a lake, ocean, river, or swimming pool. Getting some fresh air with your friends is always a good idea, but aquatic activities have a magical element that can't be explained as simply as adding two parts hydrogen and one part oxygen. Whether you canoe, paddle boat, dip in hot and cold Scandinavian baths, kayak, sail, swim, snorkel, float in a sensory deprivation tank, or sip a drink while drifting on a catamaran, Testing the Waters should indulge the urge to be in communion with that liquid wonder.

We've canoed, kayaked, and paddle-boated, but our most memorable Testing the Waters experience was in a rowboat on Devine Lake in Ontario. It was a windy August afternoon when we settled into our rowboat and drifted gently from the beach. Deb wielded one oar and Lynne had the other, and pretty soon our rowboat was spinning in circles. After experimenting with different rowing combinations, Julie—once again the steady voice of reason—determined that Lynne should take the oars while Deb navigated.

It wasn't long before the wind carried us far from shore, and the water's once-friendly demeanor became a green-eyed menace. Dark clouds gathered, and so did the search-and-rescue scenarios in our minds. Before we became the inspiration for another Gordon Lightfoot shipwreck song, we knew we had to batten down the hatches—which on a rowboat means row as if someone will batten you in the hatches if you slow down. The waves turned the minutes to hours, but we made it back to shore, a seasoned crew who wouldn't want to test the waters quite so boldly again.

If you'd prefer not to float your boat and risk an encounter with the coast guard, consider a more interactive activity. Your watery rendezvous could include a soak in a Jacuzzi or swim in a pool. A Friendly Q&A (Act 23) is the perfect activity to pair with a hot tub and beverage.

You could also participate in playful water activities with your feet firmly planted on dry land. As adults, some of us try to avoid all unnecessary encounters with water and will only allow it to touch our skin when it serves a hygienic or therapeutic purpose. But children seem to be drawn to water as if it's a transparent potion that casts a euphoric spell—a spell that seems to lose its power as we grow older. You can become enchanted again (and get a rush of endorphins) if you give yourself permission to toss a water balloon, squirt a water gun, or dance through a sprinkler. If it rains on your parade, take full advantage of the downpour and go for a walk, leaving your umbrella at home. Feel the rain on your face, stomp through the puddles instead of walking around them, and experience the delight of taking nature's shower.

As noted anthropologist and natural scientist Loren Eiseley wrote, "If there is magic on this planet, it is contained in water."

37

The Dinner of Truth

BECAUSE IF YOU THINK YOU KNOW
YOURSELF, YOU PROBABLY DON'T

"After surveying thousands of people, I've come
to the obvious but nevertheless empirically based
conclusion that one doesn't have to throw a rock
very far to hit a delusional person."

TASHA EURICH

HOW WELL DO you think you know yourself? It's a two-part
question: one part consists of how we see ourselves, the second
part is how we think others see us. So let's reframe the question: what percentage of people do you think know themselves
and how others perceive them? The answer is ten percent. Only
one person out of ten knows themselves from both an inner
and outer perspective. It's a phenomenon so rare that organiza-
tional psychologist and researcher Tasha Eurich refers to these
people as "unicorns."

We're hoping that you and your friends aren't among
the ninety percent who are delusional, but it never hurts to

double-check. And who better than your friends to tell you, in a loving way, what you need to hear? There are several acts of friendship that help you unearth who you are on the inside—from the poetic I Am From (Act 7) to the musical This Playlist Is Me (Act 24)—but The Dinner of Truth is about learning how *others* perceive you.

This activity is not for the faint of heart, which is why we have categorized it as an adventure rather than a reflection, but it is, in the truest sense, a mirroring. You give each other what you can never have, except from another person: knowledge of what you look like from the outside. Your friends have the power to help you recognize a part of yourself. This activity is well worth trying if you're brave enough to face the truth about how others see you, because it can change your life when you confront a barrier that may be holding you back.

Unfortunately, no matter how hard you try to take someone else's perspective, you will never be able to see yourself as others see you. You have to ask for help. Problem is, your friends may be reluctant to point out the metaphorical dress that you inadvertently stuffed inside the back of your panties. Do you want to know about your stuffed dress, or would you prefer to remain blissfully unaware as you roam the world accidentally exposing your underwear? What's your metaphorical dress tucked in your panties? Is it your angry aura, the way you compete with everyone over everything, or as Tasha Eurich discovered to her horror, a tendency to be high maintenance?

Now that we've sufficiently alarmed you, consider the positive: other people generally see us more accurately than we see ourselves—even strangers have an uncanny ability to size us up with only a few seconds of information, as suggested by emerging research from the University of California, Berkeley. "It's remarkable that complete strangers could pick up on who's trustworthy, kind or compassionate in twenty seconds," said lead researcher Aleksandr Kogan. Your friends can shine an even brighter light on certain aspects of yourself than strangers do, and you can choose to act on the information that they lovingly present to you. Or not.

If getting to know yourself a bit better is more important than your fear of receiving constructive feedback, then gather together a few "loving critics" for The Dinner of Truth. We can't stress enough the importance of selecting the right companions for this activity. Loving critics are friends who care deeply about you and will be honest yet gentle with their feedback. Invite only these compassionate people who have your best interests at heart to The Dinner of Truth, where food and drink are shared to make the exchange of information feel loving and comfortable rather than cold and insensitive like an employer's performance evaluation. In The Dinner of Truth, the main course is food for the soul.

Traditionally served, as described in Tasha Eurich's book *Insight*, The Dinner of Truth is where you ask your loving critic friends to tell you the one thing that annoys them most about you, and you do the same for them. You assure them that nothing is off-limits, and everyone promises to listen with an open mind.

What could possibly go wrong? Lots.

Listening without being defensive sounds good in theory, but is incredibly difficult. Especially when your fight-or-flight response kicks in and you're not thinking clearly. That's why, unless you can invite a skilled moderator such as Tasha Eurich to your gathering, we recommend an annoyance sandwich: have your friends share one thing they *love* about you before telling you the thing that annoys them, and follow it up with one more positive thing to wrap the annoyance in a delicious bun of love.

Be sure to plan this activity well in advance. Don't hit your friends with The Dinner of Truth when they think they're coming over for some wining and dining instead of toasting and roasting. Each participant should know exactly what she's signing up for—make sure all attendees read this chapter—and come prepared with the loves and annoyances written down beforehand. No one wants to intentionally blurt anything out after a couple glasses of wine. Advanced planning will give you time to think about your comments and avoid nitpicking that could lead to a tit-for-tat escalation or a not-so-loving bun fight.

When executed properly, this act of friendship can be transformative, but it's not for everyone. If it feels too risky, you can ease into The Dinner of Truth with a warm-up meal where you answer the following ten questions.

Answer these questions for yourself and for each of your friends, and compare answers:

1 What is my greatest strength?

2 What is my biggest weakness?

3 On a scale of 1 to 10, with 1 being pessimist and 10 optimist, where do I stand?

4 The one word that best describes me is...

5 The one word I wish described me is...

6 In a crisis situation I would be:

   (a) driving the ambulance;
   (b) attending to the victims;
   (c) taking selfies with a crisis backdrop;
   (d) running from the scene;
   (e) taking charge and giving orders.

7 If I had a frame around my license plate it would say, "I'd rather be [fill-in-the-blank-ing] ..."

8 When I feel uncomfortable, I...

9 My body language says I'm . . .

10 The one thing I need to work on is . . .

   You can collect anonymous responses from your friends and discuss the feedback in general, or you can take turns going around the table comparing answers to each question. The great thing about this questionnaire is that the point where what you think of yourself and what your friends think diverges will become crystal clear. If everyone else agrees on the answer to a question about you and you're the outlier, chances are you're looking at a kernel of reality. The power of The Dinner of Truth is in the *honesty* it draws out, the *reflection* it generates, and the *change* that it sparks.

38

Biker Chicks

HOP ON THE VEHICLE THAT TRANSPORTED WOMEN TO FREEDOM

"Let me tell you what I think of bicycling. I think it has done more to emancipate women than anything else in the world. I stand and rejoice every time I see a woman ride by on a wheel."
SUSAN B. ANTHONY

"SEVENTY-FIVE PERCENT OF participants will be an army of invalids within the next ten years; it brings on the most appalling diseases among young women; it swells the ranks of reckless girls and outcast women; it will prevent motherhood; and it's the devil's advance agent, morally and physically, in thousands of instances!" declared Charlotte Smith, founder of the national Women's Rescue League in the United States. What was the "it" Charlotte Smith was referring to back in the 1890s? The bicycle.

It's hard to imagine, but in the nineteenth century when the bicycle was first introduced, it was received with alarm bordering on panic. The first few women who dared to straddle the saddle of these two-wheeled wonders were trailblazers and seized the opportunity to ride away from the constraints of corsets, heavy dresses, and roles they had been stuck in for centuries. Those early women riders suffered verbal assaults and physical attacks for simply pedaling down the street without a chaperone. Little did they know they were paving the way to emancipation, the right to vote, and feminism. Sue Macy's *Wheels of Change* shares the story of this unexpected upside of the two-wheeler.

For men, it was another toy, but for women, the bicycle was the vehicle upon which they rode into a new world. It is in this spirit of discovery that we suggest you become Biker Chicks. When you go on your Biker Chicks adventure, all you'll have to endure is a butt-numbing excursion, helmet hair, and the occasional honk—a far cry from cycling in a skirt with a "mere" seven pounds of undergarments, the "rational dress" (which was once considered scandalous) of early women cyclists.

"Success in life depends as much upon a vigorous and healthy body as upon a clear and active mind," said Elsa von Blumen—one of the world's first Biker Chicks who was famous for racing her penny-farthing (also known as a high wheeler) against horses—and science is finally catching up with her. Stanford researchers are using portable MRI-like devices to try to understand how biking affects brain function, and they believe that their studies will eventually prove that cycling makes people smart and happy. Biking outdoors changes everything, as far as the brain is concerned. Stationary bikes are great for cardiovascular health, but biking on a street or trail requires continuously scanning the environment and maintaining your balance, skills that light up much more of your brain than pedaling indoors. Plus, you get the satisfaction of being outside and going somewhere.

As you prepare for your trail-blazing ride, decide if you're going to set your own course or follow an organized tour. Maps with suggested tours along bike-friendly routes are available from most bicycle rental companies. An organized bike tour is a good option if the possibility of misadventure is great (one wrong turn and you're in the bumpy part of town), or if you simply prefer to enjoy the scenery and the commentary of a knowledgeable guide rather than worry about where to find a nice ladies' room on a map. On an organized tour, you're sure to meet active people who live by the bicycle motto: "to maintain balance in life you must keep pedaling."

Search the Internet for bicycle tours in your area along with information on routes, times, cost, and, most importantly, the level of exertion. "Leisurely" and "six-hour bicycle tour" are somewhat incompatible descriptors, but don't underestimate the power of friends when they get together—your strength, endurance, and willpower will be amplified. Look for a tour with specific destinations, like a lunch spot, a beach, or a park, to break up the effort and get the endorphin rush that happens whenever you reach your goal.

You can forget about looking good in a helmet, but please don't let bicycle millinery deter you. The bold dorkiness of a bike helmet is liberating, especially when you consider that in 1895 a list of "don'ts" for women on bicycles published in *New York World* included "Don't cultivate a bicycle face" and "Don't wear a man's cap." One "don't" we can attest to is "Don't wear lip gloss," unless you enjoy turning your lips into flytraps.

We've done Biker Chicks many times and consider it to be the best way to sightsee. We biked for six hours on a guided tour through the five boroughs of New York City, a true adventure that Julie compared to giving birth. While cycling through Queens, Lynne's chain fell off the front derailleur and she became separated from the tour group, but a nice Italian tourist rescued her from a phone booth (it was 2006, before the 2007 introduction of the iPhone made cell phones appendages and the phone booth an endangered species) on a street corner with no signs. Later, during the final stage of the tour that took us through Manhattan, she fell off her bike. As Lynne's elbow hit the pavement, she couldn't decide whether to cry or not, but then recalled the fierce feminist origins of cycling and quickly recovered. You should go on a bike tour. Really.

If it's your first time back in the saddle after many years, you may set off with a bit of a wobble, but you'll relax your death grip on the handlebars soon enough, take a deep breath, and feel the gentle breeze caress your face as you realize that you truly never forget how to ride a bike. The bicycle is, to paraphrase author Iris Murdoch in her novel *The Red and the Green*, a most civilized conveyance that is pure in heart, so join your Biker Chick friends and be transported in pure joy, remembering the intrepid women who first pedaled their way to freedom.

39

The Friendly Picnic Society

LIFE IS A PICNIC WHEN YOU DINE WITH MOTHER NATURE

"There are few things so pleasant as a picnic eaten in perfect comfort."

W. SOMERSET MAUGHAM

DID YOU KNOW that the word "picnic" comes from the French word *piquenique*, which combines *piquer* (to pick or peck) and *nique* (a trifle, or a nonsense word to rhyme with *pique*)? In France, *une piquenique* referred to a group of restaurant diners who brought their own wine, but when it entered the English language in the nineteenth century, "picnic" described a fashionable party, either indoors or outdoors, to which everyone brought something to eat. The European tradition of dining outdoors predates the word picnic. Medieval hunting feasts and Renaissance country banquets were lavish, open-air affairs often associated with wealth and privilege.

The Victorian era was the golden age of picnicking. Austen and Dickens featured picnics in their plotlines, and painters such as Cézanne, Renoir, and Monet celebrated the picnic's rustic charms on canvas. In the mid-1800s, a group of Londoners developed an interesting twist on the picnic with the Picnic Society, a gathering where each person was expected to bring food and drink to share, along with some form of entertainment.

For thousands of years, long before picnics became a thing, humans hunted for food and then gathered together daily to eat outdoors. Perhaps that's why the picnic offers so many wellness benefits: we yearn to return to nature. Research tells us that being in nature can improve memory, fight depression, and lower blood pressure. In her book *The Nature Fix*, journalist Florence Williams writes that she started investigating the health benefits of nature after moving from Boulder, Colorado, to Washington, D.C., where she felt "disoriented, overwhelmed, depressed." Distilling what she learned, Williams advises us to go outside often, sometimes in wild places, and to breathe in nature with our friends.

The Friendly Picnic Society asks that you breathe in nature with your friends as you gather together for some alfresco wine and dine... and more.

A farmers' market is the ideal first stop on your picnic excursion (see Local Roots, Act 35), but in addition to food and drink, think about another element that each of you can bring to make your picnic special. You don't have to go to a lot of trouble—a Frisbee, a game, or a book of poetry is all that's needed to add a certain *je ne sais quoi* to your *piquenique*.

Location selection is critical to The Friendly Picnic Society, as nothing spoils a picnic faster than an inhospitable environment. Public parks are a good bet because they're likely to have picnic tables and benches that will give you some comfort and distance from the ants that will inevitably invite themselves to your party, but there is nothing cast in potato salad that says the society must hold all its meetings in a traditional picnic locale. Why not raise a few eyebrows and have a picnic on an accessible rooftop, at an outdoor shopping mall, or even spread a blanket, as we did, in a cemetery? (See A Grave Matter, Act 46.)

"A delightful time was had..." is how local papers often closed their write-up of an old-fashioned picnic, and it is with this wish for delightful times that we extend an invitation to you and your friends to join The Friendly Picnic Society in the hope that it will become a tradition.

40

The Tea Party Rebellion

SAVOR THIS MOST
GENTEEL ACT OF PROTEST

"She who wields a teapot has a
powerful weapon in her hand."
IRIS MACFARLANE

IT ALL BEGAN on July 9, 1848, at a party hosted by Jane Hunt,
a well-to-do New Yorker who invited four of her friends for
tea. As the women dined and sipped, they poured out their
grievances about the world's injustices toward women and, as
when 342 chests of British tea spilled into Boston Harbor and
started a revolution, a new movement was born. These five
women who came together at an afternoon tea party went on
to organize the first-ever women's rights convention at Seneca
Falls, New York. And so began the American women's suffrage
movement.

It is with this desire for righteous protest that we invite you
to join your friends in a soothing ritual steeped in history with
an aroma of revolution, The Tea Party Rebellion.

The origins of the soothing ritual known as the afternoon tea party are mysterious and theories abound, but tea historians agree that, like belly dancing, it's a uniquely feminine tradition. A reasonable fringe theory states that a mini meal with tea began as a response to the demands of organ-crushing lingerie that made it difficult to digest large meals. Another theory, discredited or simply ignored by the British, traces the tea party to the French. Most commonly, the tea party is attributed to the Duchess of Bedford, who suffered a sinking feeling around four in the afternoon and would summon her friends for "tea and a walking the fields." Whatever theory you subscribe to, having your own tea party epitomizes feminine camaraderie that nourishes your body, enriches your soul, and reminds you of your manners ... and your rights.

If you feel particularly ambitious, prepare your own afternoon tea. Do-it-yourself tea parties often feature fine china and table linens, a selection of teas—both traditional and herbal—fresh flowers, and dainty, bite-sized sandwiches and pastries. Champagne (especially pink champagne) is a welcome addition, and if the proceedings become too dainty, reading each other's tea leaves can add a note of whimsy.

But if tea party decor seems like too much of a bother, and cutting the crusts off your bread too irksome, you can do what we did and simply find a local tearoom. A hotel with a British colonial past—most major cities in North America have one—is a good place to start your search.

When we went out for afternoon tea, Lynne ordered a lavender verbena, because she said it sounded like it might be nice to bathe in. Something about tearooms makes her want to misbehave—Lynne must have been picking up on that suffragette vibe. What better place to strategize about how to make the world a better place than in the genteel oasis of a tearoom or at a tea party of your own creation?

As you bask in the tranquility of the tearoom, fortified by the company of your friends, we hope you are stirred to rebellion: What wrongs in the world do you and your friends collectively want to right? It can be anything from a desire to clean up the garbage that's littering the neighborhood, to a yearning to improve educational opportunities for women. It doesn't matter, as long as you get passionate and begin talking about all of the ways you'd like to see the world improve.

"I poured out, that day, the torrent of my long-accumulating discontent," said Elizabeth Cady Stanton, one of the invitees at Jane Hunt's fateful tea party. Her friends joined in, sharing stories of their own oppression, their inability to get an education or to vote, the expectation that they should be flawlessly subservient. Together they promised to take action, to "do and dare anything" to further their cause.

We challenge you to follow in the tea cups of these brave and passionate women who changed history. Join The Tea Party Rebellion. Find a shared cause, then do something about it.

41

Let's Go Retro!

ENTER A TIME WARP WHERE
NOTHING WILL EVER BE THE SAME

"Wherever you put the mind, the body will follow."
ELLEN LANGER

IN 1979, EIGHT men in their eighties (before eighty was the new sixty)—some stooped with arthritis, others shuffling along with canes—stepped out of a van and into 1959. As they walked through the door of a converted monastery in New Hampshire, Perry Como could be heard crooning on a radio, and Ed Sullivan welcomed them to a "really big show" on a black-and-white TV. From newspapers and magazines to food and furniture, Harvard researcher Ellen Langer designed everything to replicate the men's younger days. For five days they lived in 1959, subjects in what Langer called a "counterclockwise" study, testing the idea that wherever we put our minds, our bodies will follow.

The men were told not only to inhabit 1959, but to *become* a part of it. They were encouraged to act like the men they were twenty years ago as much as physically possible, to carry their suitcases upstairs, to do the things they enjoyed back then, and to talk about "current" events that were no longer current. After a mere five days, the results were remarkable. The men sat taller and performed better in vision, hearing, and memory tests than the control subjects who went to the monastery but were not transported back in time. Canes were cast aside and a spontaneous game of touch football broke out among the men who spent a few days living their lives like it was 1959.

And as if all that weren't enough, people who knew nothing about the study said the men *looked* younger.

In 2010, the BBC broadcast *The Young Ones* was a re-creation of Langer's study that featured six aging celebrities transported back to 1975 in all of its shag-carpeted, "Jive-Talkin'" glory. Again, test measures improved and people looked and acted younger. "I feel so much younger!" exclaimed 1970s entertainer Lionel Blair, one of the seventy-nine-year-young participants. The magic of the mind-body connection could not have been more dramatically displayed.

In Let's Go Retro! the goal is to replicate Langer's experiment to the best of your ability, with your friends. First pick a year you want to travel back in time to visit. Have everybody dress as they would have dressed back then, and bring as many artifacts from the era as possible. Cue up a playlist from that year. Watch a few TV shows from the chosen era. Play the games that used to amuse you. Eat the food that you most enjoyed. Do what we did and say goodbye to avocado toast, and hello to a jiggly Jell-O mold! As much as possible, immerse yourselves in the chosen year rather than simply reminisce about it.

Most importantly, ditch your smartphones at the door—nothing will jettison you out of a time warp and dump you back in the present moment like a news alert or a Twitter/

Facebook/Instagram scan. Let's Go Retro! is first and foremost about having fun with your friends, but it's also about observing something new about old things. Paying attention is the essence of mindfulness and how, according to Ellen Langer—whose counterclockwise study made her into an evangelist for a mindful life—we wake up, notice the wonders around us, and come to believe in the possibility of change. So travel back in time mindfully and use this activity as an opportunity to consider how it felt to live back then, and how so much about the way we look and feel is determined by our surroundings and how we think we're supposed to behave.

When your retro party is over, take some time to talk about the experience with your friends. If you traveled back to an era before smartphones, what was that like? Was there any anxiety around leaving your phone behind? How have times changed and what has remained the same? Did you find anything unpleasant about the experience? Exhilarating?

"I've been transformed!" said seventy-seven-year-old actress Sylvia Syms, who struggled to walk at the beginning of *The Young Ones* and was filmed running with her two dogs after spending a week in 1975. We hope that you discover a future of possibilities that comes from a mindful experience of the past in Let's Go Retro!

42

May I Have a Volunteer?

DO WORK THAT IS PRICELESS

"Life's most persistent and urgent question is, 'What are you doing for others?'"
MARTIN LUTHER KING JR.

DO YOU WANT to be happier, healthier, and feel like you have more time in your day? Yes? Then volunteer.

People who regularly volunteer show higher levels of happiness in their daily lives. By measuring hormones and brain activity, researchers have discovered that being helpful to others gives us immense pleasure. Human beings are hardwired to give, and the more we give, the happier we feel. According to a 2010 study from insurance company UnitedHealthcare, a whopping ninety-six percent of volunteers believe that volunteering makes them happier. Another study conducted for the U.K.'s National Council Voluntary Organisations by YouGov, a global public opinion and data company, looked at more than 10,000 volunteers who reported that volunteering improves their mental health and wellbeing, makes them feel socially connected and less isolated, and ninety percent said they feel they're making a difference. Indeed, across cultures and social classes, volunteering has been universally linked to greater quality of life and satisfaction, and lower rates of depression.

Besides lifting your mood, volunteering can improve your physical health. As Blair Lewis notes in his book *Happiness: The Real Medicine and How It Works*, a ten-year study of 2,700 men in Tecumseh, Michigan, found that those who did regular volunteer work had death rates two and a half times lower than those who didn't. Sympathetic volunteering is an example of how giving freely of your time can be doubly rewarding. For example, in Alcoholics Anonymous, where addicts with some experience in the program work with newcomers to achieve and maintain sobriety, service to others is considered an essential pillar of recovery. Similarly, recovering heart patients at Duke University Medical Center were asked to visit current heart patients to simply listen and lend support. These volunteers recovered from their heart attacks sixty percent faster than those who chose not to help other patients.

Perhaps the most surprising benefit of volunteering is the sense that you have *more* time, not less. Cassie Mogilner-Holmes, an associate professor of marketing and behavioral decision-making at UCLA's Anderson School of Management, conducted several tests and found that those who volunteer their time feel more capable, confident, and useful. Volunteers have a sense of accomplishment that makes them believe they can do more in the future. Believing that you can have an impact on the world by volunteering makes you feel like time is more abundant, and nothing is better for the soul than giving your time—your most precious, nonrenewable resource—to people in need. Help others and you will help yourself in unexpected ways. And when you volunteer with friends, the joys and benefits of giving are multiplied and the bonds of friendship are strengthened.

May I Have a Volunteer? requires some research, but it's well worth the effort. If you're extremely busy and don't want an open-ended commitment, as a group explore one-off volunteer opportunities that will involve a few hours of your time. Consider soup kitchens, senior citizens' homes, centers that support children with disabilities, women's shelters, or any organization that appeals to you. By giving your time, you'll receive a great sense of inspiration, fulfillment, and connection to people with diverse backgrounds.

It's said that the happiest people are not those who are *getting* more but those who are *giving* more. A volunteer made up the word "volunesia" to describe the moment a person forgets that they are volunteering to change lives because it's changing their own. For our May I Have a Volunteer? activity, we joined a happy, hardworking, and enthusiastic group with Habitat for Humanity on a trip to Hilton Head Island in South Carolina. Julie and Deb were assigned to cover nail heads with carpenters' caulk, a much cushier job than Lynne's sanding drywall by hand to prep for paint (but she loved the workout). We were heartened and humbled to be in the presence of people giving so much of themselves in the service of others. And, true to the research, the group at Habitat for Humanity did seem like an extraordinarily happy group of volunteers.

Beyond this friend activity, do yourself a favor and refocus your priorities to incorporate volunteering into your life. You'll be happier and healthier, and it might lead you to a different path as you explore new skills and discover that after years of working to seal the deal, you find construction work riveting.

43

Friends Immersion

EXPERIENCE A DIFFERENT WAY
OF LIFE WITHOUT THE JET LAG

"It is not our differences that divide us. It is our inability
to recognize, accept, and celebrate those differences."
AUDRE LORDE

THE IRONY WAS not lost on Esther Sternberg. Here she was,
a rheumatologist and internationally recognized expert on the
connection between stress and autoimmune disease, struck
down by inflammatory arthritis after spending several difficult years as a long-distance caregiver for her mother, who
had terminal cancer. What had been a topic of academic study
suddenly felt painfully, viscerally real.

While still deeply grieving the loss of her mother and moving into a new home, Sternberg heard a knock on the door. Her
neighbors, a Greek couple, had dropped by to welcome her to
the neighborhood with a tray of traditional Greek food. They
noticed her computer and papers strewn about and asked if
she was a writer, as they had always wanted to host one in their

cottage on the Greek island of Crete. Sternberg responded that yes, indeed, she was a writer—she was working on her first book, *The Balance Within*—and would be thrilled to join them in Crete. And so began an adventure that was to become the PBS special *The Science of Healing*. Being immersed in a different culture, seeing alternatives to the way she was living back home, would change Esther Sternberg's life for the better.

What was it about her experience in Crete that helped her heal?

"I had this 'aha' moment that what I was doing back home was all wrong," says Sternberg of her Greek epiphany. She stayed in the Cretan village of Lentas, near the ruins of the ancient temple to Asclepius, the Greek god of healing, surrounded by people of all ages who abided by the rhythms of sea and sun, grandmothers who fed her delicious, healthy Mediterranean food, and a pace of life that was much slower. Esther could relax and give herself the gift of healing through quiet contemplation, gentle physical activity, and most of all, social connection. In Crete, Sternberg was welcomed into the villagers' homes and basked in the comforting embrace of a rich network of social support that released a cascade of friendly neurochemical stress blockers.

Her exposure to life in a small Cretan village gave Sternberg an alternative to the North American lifestyle, and a set of healthy behaviors she could try out and take home with her as she continued to heal. Her example shows us how visiting a foreign land can be transformative. Esther wasn't cured of her arthritis, but her symptoms eased and the psychological shift she experienced in Crete enabled her to be at peace with herself and her illness.

You may not be able to jump on a plane to Crete with your friends, but with a little creativity you can bring a piece of Crete (or any place) into your world—it's what we call Friends

Immersion, like French immersion, but rather than language, you immerse yourselves in a culture of your choice. We'll continue with the example of Crete, since Esther Sternberg got the *keftede* (Greek meatball) rolling, but the same approach can be taken with any location that you decide you want to "visit."

To plan your event, a little research (or a lot, if you want to immerse deeply) is in order and delegation is helpful, with each friend researching a specific area of interest. With an abundance of information at your fingertips, from Wikipedia to intrepid travel author Rick Steves, never before has it been so easy to dive into a new culture. Have the audiophile among you make a playlist for your get-together based on her research into the unique music of your chosen culture—in this case, the poetic *mantinades* of Crete. Entertainment might be assigned to the most gregarious in your group. Have someone who loves to cook find recipes, while the oenophile of your group selects a regional wine, then gather everyone together to prepare some traditional food. You can make Friends Immersion into a multipart event by watching an on-point movie, such as *Zorba the Greek*, which is set on Crete and based on the book by Nikos Kazantzakis (read it, if you're a real Cretan keener); or *Little Greek Godfather*, a funny fish-out-of-water story about a little boy who travels from California to Crete for a baby's baptism.

Every culture behaves according to its own wisdom, which is often enshrined in words with no English equivalent. Prepare for Friends Immersion by having the lexophile among you—every group has one—look up a few expressions to share. Here are a few Greek words and phrases we can all learn from:

- Φιλοξενία (*filoksenia*). The first part of this word comes from the word φιλώ, or friend, while the second part comes from ξένος, stranger. It literally means "friend to the stranger" and is most often translated as "hospitality" but is much deeper than that. Hospitality is a pervasive part of Greek culture, which Esther Sternberg experienced firsthand when her new neighbors offered her food and a cottage in Crete, and the villagers of Lentas repeatedly welcomed her into their homes.

- Κέφι (*kefi*). This is the spirit of joy, passion, and enthusiasm that overwhelms the soul and requires a release in plate smashing. You can bring a little *kefi* to your Friends "Greek" Immersion with plates from the dollar store.

- Μεράκι (*meraki*). This is a word that describes the act of adding soul, creativity, and love to whatever you're doing. Be sure to add some *meraki* to all your acts of friendship.

- Για πάρτη μου (*gia party mou*). This is to do something just for you. It's almost equivalent to "treat yourself," but it's a little bit more to it than that: it's "treat yourself, and screw everything else!"

- Φιλότιμο (*filotimo*). This is the word Greeks are most proud of. The first part, as you know from the word *filoksenia*, comes from the word φιλο, or friend, and the second part comes from τιμή, meaning honor. *Filotimo* is the love of honor. It is doing what's right out of a sense of duty, regardless of the possible outcomes. *Filotimo* is also a feeling of compassion and duty toward humanity, to prioritize the well-being of others, to live for something greater than yourself.

That concludes the Greek language lesson. If you're interested in Cretan history, you'll want to find out more about the earliest known civilization of Europe, the Minoan civilization, which flourished in Crete more than four thousand years ago. And no exploration of Minoan civilization is complete without a minotaur, part man–part bull, who lived in the middle of a labyrinth.

The possibilities for an evening of labyrinthine entertainment, where together you explore the culture, food, and sensibilities of life in another land are endless. Friends Immersion is an activity that you can throw yourselves into again and again.

44

An Act of Faith

CONGREGATE IN CELEBRATION OF LIFE'S MYSTERIES

"There is only one religion, though
there are a hundred versions of it."
GEORGE BERNARD SHAW

ALL OVER THE world and in every era in history, humans have pondered the unknown. What is the meaning of life? Is there a higher power watching over our every move? Does a timeless code of moral conduct exist? Is there life after death? Does God look like Santa or Oprah? For each of these questions, there exists a religion that comforts those who believe in its answers.

Although religious intolerance continues to make horrific headlines, it's worth contemplating how much beauty religion has given the world. The creativity kindled by faith has inspired some of the world's transcendent works of art: Michelangelo's Sistine Chapel, Milton's *Paradise Lost*, da Vinci's *The Last Supper*. Religion inspired gospel music, which gave birth to the blues and rock 'n' roll. And let's not forget that Christianity isn't the only religion to make the world a better, more thoughtful, place. In 859, a young princess named Fatima al-Firhi founded the first degree-granting university in Fez, Morocco, reinforcing the importance of learning that is at the core of the Islamic tradition. Religion has enriched the lives of believers and non-believers alike. At its best, faith encourages us to embody our highest virtues, to end oppression, to forgive, and to selflessly serve others.

The *community* of worshippers who share the same beliefs and rituals is equally as important as their religious philosophy. Studies summarized by Tyler VanderWeele, professor of epidemiology at Harvard's T.H. Chan School of Public Health, have found evidence that the community and faith that religious service attendance offers is strongly associated with lower mortality, less depression, and a lower likelihood of suicide. Other health benefits found to be related to religious participation include a stronger immune system (offering some protection from drinking from a communal cup) and better cardiovascular function. Religious involvement has also been linked to higher levels of happiness and subjective wellbeing, less alcohol and drug use, lower rates of divorce, and more acts of charity. And children with a religious upbringing tend to have better mental health into adulthood.

An Act of Faith allows you to open your minds and hearts and explore a communal ritual of a faith to which each of you are unaccustomed. The presence of your friends will give you the courage to perform this activity, as it can be intimidating to enter an unfamiliar place of worship.

There are more than twenty major religions in the world, according to the "Big Religion Chart," which was created by the nondenominational website ReligionFacts, to share "just the facts" on every religion's answers to life-and-death questions. Speaking of just the facts, forty percent of Americans told Gallup that they attended church the previous weekend, yet by counting attendance at a representative sample of churches, researchers found the real number is likely closer to twenty percent. The Hartford Institute estimates that there are roughly 350,000 religious congregations in the United States with over 200 different denominations. With all this choice, a congregation out there will appeal to you and will likely be in need of attendees.

An Act of Faith is about compassionate curiosity and building your foundation of religious knowledge. The Dalai Lama wrote in the *New York Times* that, "Finding common ground among faiths can help us bridge needless divides at a time when unified action is more crucial than ever." Increasing religious literacy is one of the best ways that we can learn to live in harmony.

First, collectively decide on a religion that you want to learn more about. Do an online pilgrimage to find out more about the faith you chose and where you can experience it firsthand in your community. Next, depending on how unfamiliar the religion or community is, you may want to reach out to the organization and ask if it would be appropriate to attend a service. Or you might know someone who practices that religion and who may be able to offer an introduction. Once you're familiar with the protocols you will need to follow, and comfortable that you will be welcomed, set off for a place you've never been before to consider answers to life's mysteries.

For us, that place was the Queen Chapel African Methodist Episcopal Church in Hilton Head Island, South Carolina. The congregation welcomed us with warm smiles and open arms and asked us each to stand up, introduce ourselves, and share what churches we were visiting from. Lynne, worried that mentioning the United Church—a uniquely Canadian organization of Presbyterians and Baptists—would sound like she worshipped an airline, decided to go with Presbyterian. After the introductions, we sang along to gospel music, listened to a touching Father's Day sermon, and left feeling uplifted. We were reminded of all the good religion does to bring people together, bond them in shared emotion, and offer a salve for the world's injustices.

In his essay "Meditation in a Toolshed," British author C.S. Lewis said that we will gain greater insight into other belief systems by stepping inside and looking "along" with them as a lived experience, rather than looking "at" them from the outside. Looking "along," 143 leaders from all the major faiths signed a declaration at the 1993 Parliament of the World's Religions: "We must treat others as we wish others to treat us."

Amen.

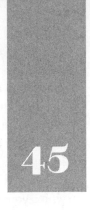

45

Live and Let's Learn

BEING INTERESTING STARTS
WITH BEING INTERESTED

"Live as if you were to die tomorrow.
Learn as if you were to live forever."
MAHATMA GANDHI

AS REPORTED BY BBC News, Priscilla Sitienei, a midwife from rural Kenya, had never learned to read or write, but she wanted to capture the story of her life because she wanted to share the lessons of her experience. So at age ninety, Priscilla went to school along with six of her great-great grandchildren. "I want to say to the children of the world, especially girls, that education will be your wealth," Priscilla says.

We can blame Aristotle for our lingering "can't-teach-an-old-dog-new-tricks" mentality that caused many potential Priscillas to hesitate to learn what they've always wanted to learn, or even to trust their memory when a GPS is at hand. Aristotle believed the young mind was a tablet made of hot wax on which learning could easily form an impression. Over time, the wax of the mind becomes cold and brittle, making imprinting new knowledge almost impossible.

But the latest research into neuroplasticity—the ability of the brain to remake itself—encourages us to keep on learning: it's never too late to pick up a new skill, behavior, or subject. Learning is especially easy if you exercise (see Move Ya Body, Act 34), which generates new brain cells—fresh, hot cranial wax on which you can imprint new information. And according to a MacArthur Foundation study that focused on lifestyle factors that contribute to successful aging, three things can prevent age-related cognitive decline: maintaining an optimal weight, exercising, and engaging in continuous learning. Science has finally caught up with Plato, who more than two millennia ago said that through education and physical activity we can attain perfection. Perhaps he was overselling continuous learning a bit, but according to Ipsit Vahia, director of geriatric outpatient services for Harvard-affiliated McLean Hospital, "The same concept applies to the brain [as the body]. You need to exercise it with new challenges to keep it healthy."

Learning keeps your brain nimble and it also makes you happy. As Columbia University professor Andrew Delbanco says, learning enables you to "shape a life that leads you to a happy place." And, according to research cited in the *Harvard Business Review*, when it comes to dealing with stress, learning something new is even better than relaxation.

To achieve the stress-busting benefits from learning, you need the fuel that drives the urge to learn: curiosity. Curiosity is becoming a widely recognized business superpower. Some of the world's most successful people are also the most curious; they have what scientists refer to as "a drive state for information," which can also be observed in organisms as simple as roundworms. Jeff Bezos, founder of Amazon, taps into his curiosity in an intentional way to enliven his life and his business. In her 2018 commencement speech, Oprah Winfrey wished

University of Southern California students "curiosity and confidence." SpaceX CEO Elon Musk had such a curious mind that he taught himself rocket science. All great businesspeople have insatiable, yet intentional, curiosity. Too much unfocused curiosity and you get an unsettled "butterfly mind" that never lingers long enough on a single topic to make the information useful; too little curiosity and you become a roundworm, your interest limited to only the information necessary for basic survival.

Curiosity has an underappreciated role in wellbeing: there is much in life that you can't control, but you can always cultivate a curious mind. Susan Noonan, psychologist and author of *Managing Your Depression*, calls curiosity the "big life preserver" that pulls you into the flow of life and out of depression. According to research reported by BBC Capital, an interest in new ideas has many advantages and is a key characteristic of the highly promotable "high-potential personality." Curiosity makes you more creative, enables you to learn more easily, and protects you from burnout. You can add CQ, the curiosity quotient, to EQ, the emotional intelligence quotient, because a passion to learn and be curious will spill over into your relationships. Have you ever had conversations with incurious people who are content to talk about themselves and show no interest in anyone or anything else, making small talk feel especially claustrophobic? Being genuinely interested in learning about (and from) others will make you instantly likeable and the rock star of any gathering. Live and Let's Learn draws on your CQ and asks you to ask yourself two questions: (a) What am I curious to know more about? and (b) What can I teach my friends?

Do you have a yearning to learn about artificial intelligence? Life on Mars? It doesn't have to be something earth-shattering or interplanetary. Lynne would simply like to learn how to apply smoky-eye makeup without looking like she's been punched in the face (seriously, after watching a video and painstakingly following its paint-by-numbers instructions, someone asked her if she'd been attacked).

In 2018, the professional basketball team the Philadelphia 76ers experienced an incredible turnaround that was attributed in part to a culture of continuous learning: during breakfast meetings players would share information on topics from coffee to snakes, from tattoos to simulation theory, to anything that piqued their curiosity. Teaching is a great way to bolster your own knowledge, and you'll gain a deeper and longer-lasting understanding of a topic when you share it with others through a phenomenon known as the "protégé effect." In a study out of the University of Georgia, students who taught other students increased their understanding of the material by two letter grades. So you can jump from a "C" grade understanding of a topic to a "B+" or even an "A-" by teaching it.

Follow these three simple steps and you'll reap the benefits of learning something new, exercising your brain, and improving the mental, emotional, and cognitive health of your friends.

Each of you should answer the questions yourself and then circulate your answers amongst your friends:

1 **Write down three topics that pique your interest.** Don't choose anything overwhelming like quantum physics. Try a bite-sized topic—something like meatless meat—that won't take a lot of time to research to satisfy your curiosity, and straightforward enough that you can learn a lot about it quickly and confidently share your newfound knowledge with your friends.

2 **Write down three topics in which you're qualified to share your expertise.** Here are some ideas to consider:

   • Are you a cook extraordinaire? Channel your inner Julia Child and teach your friends an easy, impressive dish.

- Do you know another language? Give friends a few handy phrases to practice.

- Can you play an instrument? Teach your friends a few chords.

- Are you an artsy type? Show your friends a painting, sculpting, or photography technique.

- Do you know how to dance? Teach your friends a few of your favorite moves.

- Is there a book you've read that you'd like to summarize for your friends?

3 **Choose a topic to present.** Of the six topics you've written down—three areas of interest and three areas of expertise—select one for a brief presentation to your friends (or if you can't decide on a topic, have your friends choose one for you based on their interest).

Make your presentation fun and entertaining by using creative formats like PowerPoint or a flip chart or, if you've always wanted to star in a documentary, record a YouTube video on the topic to share with your friends. Using a game setup like *Jeopardy!* or Trivial Pursuit can make even dull topics (not that yours will be dull) come to life.

And if nobody has the time or energy for a presentation or documentary production, you can still do the activity Live and Let's Learn. Never before in history has it been so easy to learn so much from so many in so little time. Online courses abound—many of which are free. Do you have any idea how much it would cost to invite a high-profile guest speaker to your next get-together? Any professional worth listening to typically charges a speaker's fee that would exceed most potluck budgets.

But there is a way to have a notable expert entertain you with a lecture on topics as diverse as spaghetti sauce (see Malcolm Gladwell's "Choice, Happiness and Spaghetti Sauce") and orgasms (see Mary Roach's: "10 Things You Didn't Know about Orgasm"). We highly recommend Robert Waldinger's "What Makes a Good Life? Lessons from the Longest Study on Happiness" because it stresses the importance and connectivity of relationships to wellbeing. Simply fire up your laptop, hook it up to your television, and go to TED.com. Choose from a menu of hundreds of speeches, and in an instant you will have a free twenty-minute keynote address that is certain to generate plenty of intellectual sparks. Talks at Google, commencement speeches, and podcasts are other great sources of keynotes for your next friendly get-together.

Let learning enliven and enrich you.

46

A Grave Matter

NOTHING MAKES YOU FEEL MORE ALIVE THAN A VISIT TO THE CEMETERY

"She did it the hard way."

BETTE DAVIS' EPITAPH

DID YOU KNOW that the living room used to be known as the death room? Victorian etiquette called for properly and publicly mourning loved ones, which meant displaying the deceased in the parlor along with their clothing, jewelry, and other personal items. Medical practices of the nineteenth century weren't sophisticated enough to always accurately determine death, so the body was closely observed for a few days to make sure the corpse didn't suddenly awaken, horror-movie style, following a long sleep or illness. Thus we have the word "wake" to describe ritual visitation of the deceased before the burial.

Once medical professionals could officially confirm death, bodies were moved to funeral homes and death rooms became living rooms. Around the same time, graveyards moved from urban to rural settings, a change of scene that reflected the

Romantic era's love of nature. Far from creepy or depressing, the first cemeteries were conceived as beautiful public parks where people would gather for picnics and children would play. A natural setting far removed from the busy, noisy, unfeeling space of the city was believed to be conducive to a heightened state of peace and reflection.

As our culture became increasingly focused on celebrating youth and vitality, and local green space that didn't include dead people became more abundant, cemeteries started to be perceived as creepier locales. But times are changing for taphophiles—people who love cemeteries—and those with a curiosity about the past. The rising popularity of genealogy along with a cultural shift toward embracing the cemetery's roots as a public space is making the graveyard once again a popular gathering place. You can attend a yoga class at Laurel Hill Cemetery in Philadelphia. Michigan Memorial Park cemetery in Flat Rock holds fishing derbies in its pond. And, befitting its name, Hollywood Forever Cemetery holds movie nights and once hosted a concert by Lana Del Rey, who must have sung one of her deadliest songs, "Born to Die."

Hopefully, now that you know more about cemeteries, we have convinced you to at least consider visiting one with your friends so that together you can think about life in its richness and mystery, and perhaps, as we did, even enjoy a picnic. Visiting a graveyard needn't be a solemn experience and can be enlivened by a bit of research beforehand: look into its history, its notable inhabitants, and the stories it has to tell. Think of A Grave Matter as a trip to an outdoor natural history museum, or the viewing of a collection of personalized sculptures with inscriptions describing what was most important to people of a particular time and place.

Some cemeteries are the final resting places of famous people, others have tombstones with interesting epitaphs, but all graveyards offer a quiet, soulful experience to contemplate the dashes between dates of birth and death. Every stone is a life, a story. And, according to a study of "mortality salience," you'll find some generous people there: after their visits, people who go to cemeteries are more likely to help others than those who simply walked in the vicinity of one.

We were fortunate to be able to visit one of the most visually stunning cemeteries in the world, the famed Bonaventure Cemetery in Savannah, Georgia. In preparation for our visit, we read John Berendt's book *Midnight in the Garden of Good and Evil*, which featured the Bonaventure Cemetery on its cover. Although there were thousands of graves and we didn't have a map to guide us, we stumbled—thankfully not literally—on many of the plots mentioned in the book, including those of Johnny Mercer and Pulitzer Prize–winning poet Conrad Aiken and his parents.

The finality of so many lives in one place will hopefully encourage you to reflect on your past and to ponder your future. When you're suspended between death, nature, and the bustle of everyday life, take advantage of the stillness of the cemetery and allow it to speak to you. Listen hard. And if you're up for it, consider writing your own epitaph and inviting your friends to do likewise.

Deb's epitaph: *She took the stairway to heaven.*

Lynne's epitaph: *Workout complete.*

Julie's epitaph: *I'll be back . . .*

47

Put Slumber Back in the Party

REBEL AGAINST A HEALTHY BEDTIME ROUTINE, BUT JUST THIS ONCE

"The older you get, the fewer slumber parties there are, and I hate that. I liked slumber parties. What happened to them?"

DREW BARRYMORE

PUT SLUMBER BACK in the Party is less ambitious (and much less expensive) than a "girlfriend getaway," and more intensive than a quick lunch or coffee, but is guaranteed to add some fun to your friendly get-together and deepen your relationships. Adult slumber parties are officially a thing, featured in *Washington Post* headlines as well as Dua Lipa's video for her song "New Rules." Even museums are getting into the slumber party trend, with the Natural History Museum in London offering "Dino Snores for Grown-ups," a sleepover for people who aren't afraid of dinosaur skeletons coming to life in the middle of the night.

This book is brimming with fun things you can do at your slumber party—we highly recommend A Friendly Q&A (Act 23)—

but for a moment we'd like to take the focus off the *party* and look at the *slumber*, or rather the deficit of it.

Insufficient sleep makes you forgetful, impulsive, moody, unable to learn new things, more prone to dementia, more likely to die of a heart attack, less able to fend off sickness with a strong immune system, and it makes your body hurt more. It also messes with your genes and increases your risk of death due to accidents. There's nothing more important for your physical *and* mental health than adequate sleep, which for the overwhelming majority of adults means eight hours per night.

It's called "beauty sleep" for a reason—a good night's sleep is the key for a radiant complexion. As you slumber, your blood flow increases and your body makes new collagen, which plumps up your skin and helps fade wrinkles and the dark circles under your eyes. Studies have shown that people who get insufficient sleep are perceived as less attractive than their well-rested counterparts. But the need for sleep goes far beyond beauty.

The Centers for Disease Control and Prevention reported that more than a third of American adults don't get enough sleep, and women are twice as likely as men to suffer from insomnia. Why would we be designed to spend a third of our lives snoozing, a vulnerable position for our ancient ancestors who slept outdoors among the critters, unless what's happening to our bodies while we sleep is a nonnegotiable biological necessity? While we sleep it may appear as though we're being unproductive—hence the culture of "you snooze, you lose"— but our sleeping bodies are busy, busy, busy. Think of sleep as the time when you receive a visit from a high-tech specialist in life-support systems. This nocturnal visitor sweeps away the debris of the day that has been clogging up your brain, organizes new learning, and fortifies your defenses against invading organisms. Let's call this diligent worker "Ms. Sandman," who has a critical job description that we underappreciate at our peril.

The first thing Ms. Sandman does once you're asleep is lower your blood pressure to give your heart a break. Then she releases hormones that promote tissue growth to help heal injuries, sore muscles, and inflammation. A check of your metabolic system tells her how much ghrelin and leptin are required. Ghrelin is the hormone that triggers hunger and leptin is the hormone that tells you when you're full. If Ms. Sandman doesn't have time to do her job properly, you'll crave sweets and find it hard to stop after the first cookie. A study in the *European Journal of Clinical Nutrition* showed that people ate an average of nearly 385 more calories per day when they were in a state of sleep deprivation because they were less able to control their appetites. Before Ms. Sandman leaves, she makes more white blood cells for your arsenal to attack viruses and bacteria. In another study, this one led by Sheldon Cohen, professor of psychology at Carnegie Mellon University, people who slept for at least eight hours were three times less likely to catch a cold than people who got seven hours or less.

This is only a fraction of Ms. Sandman's job description, which also includes cleansing the brain of plaque buildup that can lead to Alzheimer's disease and directing the activity of killer cells that target cancer.

Ms. Sandman has a vital role and she needs eight hours to do it properly. So how can we help her?

Here's our handy mnemonic, based on expert advice, for REST:

- **Routine.** Go to bed at the same time every night at an hour when you feel tired, and get out of bed at roughly the same time every morning. Even on weekends. Consistency is critical to good sleep hygiene. Ms. Sandman doesn't like it when you mess with her work schedule. But she does like it when you welcome her with a wind-down ritual that involves things like a warm bath, a few moments of reflection on the highlights of the day, a meditation, or a print (not electronic) book. She doesn't mind sex either, as long as it's good.

- **Exercise.** A substantial body of evidence suggests that exercise improves sleep, providing it's not within four hours of bedtime. Physical activity can increase the time spent in deep sleep, the most physically restorative sleep phase. Exercise also increases sleep duration, reduces stress and anxiety, and is an effective therapy for insomnia and other sleep disorders like sleep apnea.

- **Stop eating after dinner.** Avoid heavy meals, caffeine, and excessive alcohol too close to bedtime. You may be unable to resist the allure of a nightly snack, but try not to eat anything at least two hours before going to bed.

- **Turn off technology.** Not only is it important to turn off the computer at least an hour before bedtime, but don't do any work or watch a program that might stimulate your mind in a way that makes it hard to wind down. For heaven's sake, don't watch or listen to the news before bed! Ms. Sandman can't stand it when she has to listen to nightmares while she works.

Your slumber party will likely break at least one REST rule, but if you spend a few minutes talking about sleep with your friends, sharing your wind-down routines, and encouraging one another to get eight hours, Ms. Sandman will forgive you this once.

Put Slumber Back in the Party includes a celebration, and we have a few suggestions based on our extensive slumber party experience. Hosting a sleepover shouldn't require wielding a spiralizer, dehydrator, or thermal immersion circulator. Pizza and munchies or anything informal that might be described as "eats" set the perfect mood; however, you can add a touch elegance to the event with a dress code of fancy pajamas. With hours to spend together, you can deepen your conversation and move beyond the superficial chitchat and get to what's *really* going on in your lives. The struggles, the triumphs, the laughs, and the tears will all pour out as the lights dim and everyone feels illuminated by acts of friendship.

You may not get the required eight hours of sleep at your slumber party, but the benefits of investing in your closest relationships are worth it.

Acknowledgments

WE WOULD LIKE to thank all of the women out there who inspire other women grow through encouragement, love, and support. You make the world a better place.

To everyone at Page Two, thank you for guiding us through this journey, especially our talented editor Kendra Ward, who helped us make *Acts of Friendship* the best version of itself; and Page Two co-founder Trena White, who saw potential in a book with a powerful message. Shout outs also go to Peter Cocking and his design team, who wrapped our work in a striking package; Annemarie Tempelman-Kluit, who helped us channel our enthusiasm into a strategic marketing plan; and proofreader extraordinaire, Alison Strobel.

A dear friend once told Lynne something she will never forget: "We're so lucky to be surrounded by angels." Lynne thanks all the angels in her life: friends, family, and especially her husband, Louie, whose love helps her flourish. She is grateful for angelic co-authors Deb Mangolt and Julie Smethurst and thanks them for their love, enthusiasm, wise insights, and compassion that have truly made her a better person.

Deb thanks her husband, Randy, for his never-ending love and for being supportive of absolutely everything she wants to do; friends and family, whose daily acts of friendship fill her with love and gratitude; and Lynne and Julie for showing her that we can learn from our friends and help each other become better versions of ourselves.

Julie thanks her husband, Bill, for believing in her and for helping make her dreams come true; her children Geoff, Rachel, and Brad for bringing endless love, joy, and lessons to her life; and all the others that she loves, especially Alison, Charlie, and Adelynn for making life so wonderful. Lynne and Deb's friendship has guided Julie along her journey so far, and hopefully will continue to do so for many years to come. Much love to you both.

Resources

THE FOLLOWING PUBLICATIONS and other media resources served as sources and inspiration for the activities in this book. We hope, dear friends, that should you wish to pursue the art and science of friendship, health, and wellbeing any further, that these provide you with a rich start.

Before the First Act

Holt-Lunstad, Julianne, Timothy B. Smith, and J. Bradley Layton. "Social Relationships and Mortality Risk: A Meta-analytic Review." *PloS Med* 7, no. 7 (2010): e1000316. https://doi.org/10.1371/journal .pmed.1000316.

McPherson, Miller, Lynn Smith-Lovin, and Matthew E. Brashears. "Social Isolation in America: Changes in Core Discussion Networks over Two Decades." *American Sociological Review* 71 (2006): 353–75. https:// doi.org/10.1177/000312240607100301.

Mineo, Liz. "Good Genes Are Nice, but Joy Is Better." *The Harvard Gazette,* April 11, 2017. https://news.harvard.edu/gazette/story/2017/04/ over-nearly-80-years-harvard-study-has-been-showing-how-to-live- a-healthy-and-happy-life/.

Morris, Margaret E., and Sherry Turkle. *Left to Our Own Devices: Outsmarting Smart Technology to Reclaim Our Relationships, Health, and Focus.* Cambridge, MA: Massachusetts Institute of Technology, 2018.

Nelson, Shasta. *Frientimacy: How to Deepen Friendships for Lifelong Health and Happiness*. Berkeley, CA: Seal Press, 2016.

Olds, Jacqueline, and Richard Schwartz. *The Lonely American: Drifting Apart in the Twenty-First Century*. Boston: Beacon Press, 2009.

Turkle, Sherry. *Alone Together: Why We Expect More from Technology and Less from Each Other*. New York: Basic Books, 2012.

———. *Reclaiming Conversation: The Power of Talk in a Digital Age*. New York: Penguin, 2015.

Vaillant, George. *Aging Well: Surprising Guideposts to a Happier Life from the Landmark Study of Adult Development*. New York: Little, Brown and Company, 2003.

———. *Triumphs of Experience: The Men of the Harvard Grant Study*. Cambridge: Belknap Press, 2015.

1. Take Your Cue

Alimujiang, Aliya, Ashley Wiensch, Jonathan Boss, Nancy L. Fleischer, Alison M. Mondul, Karen McLean, Bhramar Mukherjee, and Celeste Leigh Pearce. "Association between Life Purpose and Mortality among U.S. Adults Older Than 50 Years." *Journal of the American Medical Association Network Open* 2, no. 5 (2019): e194270. https://jamanetwork.com/journals/jamanetworkopen/fullarticle/2734064.

Campbell, Joseph. *The Power of Myth*. New York: First Anchor Books, 1991.

García, Héctor, and Francesc Miralles. *Ikigai: The Japanese Secret to a Long and Happy Life*. New York: Penguin, 2017.

Gordon, Mara. "Having a Sense of Purpose Is Linked to Health." NPR (website), May 25, 2019. https://www.npr.org/sections/health-shots/2019/05/25/726695968/whats-your-purpose-finding-a-sense-of-meaning-in-life-is-linked-to-health.

Rankin, Lissa. "The Shocking Truth about Our Health." Filmed 2011. TEDxFiDiWomen video, 18:02. https://www.youtube.com/watch?v=7tu9nJmr4xs&feature=youtu.be.

———. *Your Inner Pilot Light: Connecting with the Infinite Source of Love, Guidance, and Healing*. Read by the author. Louisville, CO: Sounds True, 2018. Audible audio ed., 8 hr., 45 min.

2. The Chuck-It List

Ware, Bronnie. *The Top Five Regrets of the Dying—A Life Transformed by the Dearly Departing*. London: Hay House, 2011.

3. Brag Queens

McKee, Annie. *How to Be Happy at Work: The Power of Purpose, Hope, and Friendship*. Boston: Harvard Business Review Press, 2018.

Montague, Charlotte. *Women of Invention: Life-Changing Ideas by Remarkable Women*. New York: Chartwell Books, 2018.

Russo, Nicholas P. "Margaret Hamilton, Apollo Software Engineer, Awarded Presidential Medal of Freedom." *NASA History*, November 2016. https://www.nasa.gov/feature/margaret-hamilton-apollo-software-engineer-awarded-presidential-medal-of-freedom.

Silva, Christine, and Nancy Carter. "Women Don't Go After the Big Jobs with Gusto: True or False?" *Harvard Business Review*, October 2011. https://hbr.org/2011/10/women-dont-go-after-the-big-job.

4. A Senseless Dinner

Albers, Susan, and Lilian Cheung. *Eating Mindfully: How to End Mindless Eating and Enjoy a Balanced Relationship with Food*. Oakland: New Harbinger Publications, 2012.

Chozen Bays, Jan. "Mindful Eating." *Psychology Today*, February 5, 2009. https://www.psychologytoday.com/us/blog/mindful-eating/200902/mindful-eating.

De Castro, J.M. "Family and Friends Produce Greater Social Facilitation of Food Intake Than Other Companions." *Physiology and Behavior* 56, no. 3 (1994): 445–50.

Hanh, Thich Nhat. *How to Eat (Mindfulness Essentials)*. Berkeley: Parallax Press, 2014.

Hanh, Thich Nhat, and Lilian Cheung. *Savor: Mindful Eating, Mindful Life*. New York: HarperOne, 2011.

Kabat-Zinn, John. *Coming to Our Senses: Healing Ourselves and the World through Mindfulness*. New York: Hachette Books, 2006.

Morgan, Richard. "Brooklyn Foodies Supper in Silence." *Wall Street Journal*, September 17, 2013. https://blogs.wsj.com/metropolis/2013/09/17/brooklyn-foodies-supper-in-silence/.

Neuroscience News. "An On-Off Switch for Brain Plasticity following Vision Loss," *NeuroscienceNews.com*, August 12, 2015. https://neurosciencenews.com/neuroplasticity-vision-loss-2420/.

5. A Journal of Discovery

Cameron, Julia. *The Artist's Way: 25th Anniversary Edition*. New York: TarcherPerigee, 2016.

Frank, Anne. *The Diary of a Young Girl*. New York: Bantam Books, 1993.

Pennebaker, James W., and John F. Evans. *Expressive Writing: Words That Heal*. Enumclaw, WA: Idyll Arbor, 2014.

Smyth, Joshua M., Arthur Stone, Adam Hurewitz, and Alan Kaell. "Effects of Writing about Stressful Experiences on Symptom Reduction in Patients with Asthma or Rheumatoid Arthritis." *Journal of the American Medical Association* 281, no. 14 (1999): 1304-9. https://www.ncbi.nlm.nih.gov/pubmed/10208146.

6. Childhood Excavations

Addis, Donna Rose, Alana T. Wong, and Daniel L. Schacter. "Remembering the Past and Imagining the Future: Common and Distinct Neural Substrates during Event Construction and Elaboration." *Neuropsychologia* 45 (2007): 1363-77. https://www.ncbi.nlm.nih.gov/pubmed/17126370.

Ban Breathnach, Sarah. *Something More: Excavating Your Authentic Self*. New York: Grand Central Publishing, 2000.

Irish, M., D.R. Addis, J.R. Hodges, and O. Piguet. "Considering the Role of Semantic Memory in Episodic Future Thinking: Evidence from Semantic Dementia." *Brain* 135, no. 7 (2012): 2178-91. https://www.ncbi.nlm.nih.gov/pubmed/22614246.

7. I Am From

Zapruder, Matthew. *Why Poetry*. New York: Ecco, 2017.

And four excellent resources for poems to read out loud:

Dickinson, Emily. *The Essential Emily Dickinson*. Selected and with an introduction by Joyce Carol Oates. New York: Ecco, 2016.

Oliver, Mary. *Devotions: The Selected Poems of Mary Oliver*. New York: Penguin Press, 2017.

Pinsky, Robert. *Essential Pleasures: A New Anthology of Poems to Read Aloud*. New York: W.W. Norton, 2009.

Rich, Adrienne. *Arts of the Possible: Essays and Conversations*. New York: W.W. Norton, 2001.

8. Moments of Meditation

Barbor, Cary. "The Science of Meditation." *Psychology Today*, May 1, 2001. https://www.psychologytoday.com/ca/articles/200105/the-science-meditation.

Brach, Tara. *Radical Acceptance: Embracing Your Life with the Heart of a Buddha*. New York: Bantam Dell, 2003. *(Tara Brach offers a wide range of guided meditations and lectures, for an optional donation, on her website: www.tarabrach.com.)*

Hölzel, Britta, James Carmody, Mark Vangel, Christina Congleton, Sita M. Yerramseti, Tim Gard, and Sara W. Lazar. "Mindfulness Practice Leads to Increases in Regional Brain Gray Matter Density." *Psychiatry Research: Neuroimaging* 191, no. 1 (2011): 36–9. https://www.ncbi.nlm.nih.gov/pmc/articles/PMC3004979/.

Lazar, Sara. "How Meditation Can Reshape Our Brains." TEDxCambridge. Filmed 2011, Cambridge Massachusetts, 8:33. https://www.youtube.com/watch?v=m8rRzTtP7Tc.

McGreevey, Sue. "Eight Weeks to a Better Brain." *Harvard Gazette*, January 21, 2011. https://news.harvard.edu/gazette/story/2011/01/eight-weeks-to-a-better-brain/.

Neff, Kristin, and Christopher Germer. "A Pilot Study and Randomized Controlled Trial of the Mindful Self-Compassion Program." *Journal of Clinical Psychology* 69, no. 1 (2013): 28–44. https://www.ncbi.nlm.nih.gov/pubmed/23070875. *(Kristin Neff has a selection of guided self-compassion meditations on her website: https://self-compassion.org.)*

Salzberg, Sharon. *Lovingkindness: The Revolutionary Art of Happiness*. Berkeley: Shambhala, 2002.

9. To Give Is to Receive

Baraz, James, and Shoshana Alexander. "The Helper's High." *Greater Good Magazine*, February 1, 2010. https://greatergood.berkeley.edu/article/item/the_helpers_high.

Bea, Scott. "Wanna Give? This Is Your Brain on a 'Helper's High.'" *Cleveland Clinic*, November 2016. https://health.clevelandclinic.org/why-giving-is-good-for-your-health/.

Piferi, Rachel L., and Kathleen A. Lawler. "Social Support and Ambulatory Blood Pressure: An Examination of Both Giving and Receiving." *International Journal of Psychophysiology* 62, no. 2 (2006): 328–36. https://doi.org/10.1016/j.ijpsycho.2006.06.002.

Post, Stephen, and Jill Neimark. *Why Good Things Happen to Good People: How to Live a Longer, Healthier, Happier Life by the Simple Act of Giving.* New York: Broadway Books, 2008.

10. Mock Therapy

Berk, Lee S., Stanley A. Tan, William F. Fry, Barbara J. Napier, Jerry W. Lee, Richard W. Hubbard, John E. Lewis, and William C. Eby. "Neuroendocrine and Stress Hormone Changes during Mirthful Laughter." *American Journal of the Medical Sciences* 298, no. 6 (1989): 390–6. https://www.ncbi.nlm.nih.gov/pubmed/2556917.

Mayo Clinic Staff. "Stress Relief from Laughter? It's No Joke." Mayo Clinic (website). April 2019. https://www.mayoclinic.org/healthy-lifestyle/stress-management/in-depth/stress-relief/art-20044456.

Python Pictures. *Monty Python and the Holy Grail.* Burbank, California: RCA/Columbia Pictures Home Video, 1991.

Savage, Brandon, Heidi Lujan, Raghavendar Thipparthi, and Stephen DiCarlo. "Humor, Laughter, Learning, and Health! A Brief Review." *Advances in Physiology Education* 41, no. 3 (2017): 341–7. https://www.ncbi.nlm.nih.gov/pubmed/28679569.

11. Thank You, Thank You, Thank You

Emmons, Robert. *Thanks!: How Practicing Gratitude Can Make You Happier.* New York: Houghton Mifflin, 2008.

Emmons, Robert, and Michael E. McCullough. "Counting Blessings versus Burdens: An Experimental Investigation of Gratitude and Subjective Well-Being in Daily Life." *Journal of Personality and Social Psychology* 84, no. 2 (2003): 377–89. https://www.researchgate.net/publication/325698475.

Emmons, Robert, and Robin Stern. "Gratitude as a Psychotherapeutic Intervention." *Journal of Clinical Psychology* 69, no. 8 (2013):846–55. http://ei.yale.edu/wp-content/uploads/2013/11/jclp22020.pdf.

Marsh, Jason. "Tips for Keeping a Gratitude Journal." *Greater Good Magazine*, November 17, 2011. https://greatergood.berkeley.edu/article/item/tips_for_keeping_a_gratitude_journal.

Sood, Amit. *The Mayo Clinic Handbook for Happiness: A 4-Step Plan for Resilient Living*. Boston: Da Capo Lifelong Books, 2015.

12. Forgive and Hike On

Hari, Johann. *Lost Connections: Why You're Depressed and How to Find Hope*. New York: Bloomsbury, 2018.

Herrera, Tim. "Let Go of Your Grudges. They're Doing You No Good." *New York Times*, May 2019. https://www.nytimes.com/2019/05/19/smarter-living/let-go-of-your-grudges-theyre-doing-you-no-good.html.

Luskin, Fred. Forgive For Good (website). https://learningtoforgive.com.

Mayo Clinic Staff. "Forgiveness: Letting Go of Grudges and Bitterness." Mayo Clinic (website), November 2017. https://www.mayoclinic.org/healthy-lifestyle/adult-health/in-depth/forgiveness/art-20047692.

13. It's Easy Being Green

Associated Press. "Best Way to Fight Climate Change? Plant a Trillion Trees." CBC News (website). July 5, 2019. https://www.cbc.ca/news/technology/tree-planting-climate-change-1.5201102.

NASA. "Climate Change: How Do We Know?" NASA Global Climate Change (website). Updated June 20, 2019. https://climate.nasa.gov/evidence/.

Suckling, James, and Jacquetta Lee. "Redefining Scope: The True Environmental Impact of Smartphones?" *International Journal of Life Cycle Assessment* 20, no. 8 (2015): 1181–96. https://www.researchgate.net/publication/277996263.

14. A Friendly Multiple-Choice Quiz

Mayo Clinic Staff. "Friendships: Enrich Your Life and Improve Your Health." Mayo Clinic (website). September 28, 2016. https://www.mayoclinic.org/healthy-lifestyle/adult-health/in-depth/friendships/art-20044860.

15. A Woman's Rite

Angelou, Maya. *Phenomenal Woman: Four Poems Celebrating Women*. New York: Random House, 1994.

Artspace Editors. "Oh My Goddess! 8 Ancient Female Deities from Art History." Artspace (website). October 8, 2015. https://www.artspace .com/magazine/art_101/book_report/phaidon-goddess-list-53182.

Campbell, Joseph. *Goddesses: Mysteries of the Feminine Divine*. Oakland: New World Library, 2013.

Eneix, Linda. "Of Temples and Goddesses in Malta." *Popular Archaeology*, February 6, 2011. https://popular-archaeology.com/article/of-temples-and-goddesses-in-malta/.

Estés, Clarissa Pinkola. *Women Who Run with the Wolves: Myths and Stories of the Wild Woman Archetype*. New York: Ballantine Books, 1996.

Marsden, Harriet. "International Women's Day: What Are Matriarchies, and Where Are They Now?" *Independent*, March 8, 2018. https://www .independent.co.uk/news/long_reads/international-womens-day-matriarchy-matriarchal-society-women-feminism-culture-matrilineal-elephant-a8243046.html.

16. Think on Your Stilettos

Abrahams, Matt. *Speaking Up without Freaking Out: 50 Techniques for Confident and Compelling Presenting*. Dubuque, IA: Kendall Hunt Publishing Company, 2016.

Donovan, Jeremey. *How to Win the World Championship of Public Speaking*. Self-published, CreateSpace Independent Publishing Platform, 2013.

Zekeri, Andrew. "College Curriculum Competencies and Skills Former Students Found Essential to Their Careers." *College Student Journal* 38, no. 3 (2004): 412–34. https://eric.ed.gov/?id=EJ706689.

And a video to inspire your own quick thinking:

Rothschild, Connor. "Was the U.S. War in Afghanistan in Vain?" Filmed 2017. JenniferRothschild, 10:40. https://www.youtube.com/watch?v=lzoUu1fDmWE. *(A young competitor at the 2017 International Extemporaneous Speaking National Championship.)*

17. Get On Board

Farber, Neil. "Throw Away Your Vision Board: Vision Boards Are for Dreaming, Action Boards Are for Achieving." *Psychology Today*, May 23, 2012. https://www.psychologytoday.com/ca/blog/the-blame-game/201205/throw-away-your-vision-board-0.

Ranganathan, Vinoth, Vlodek Siemionow, Jingzhi Liu, Vinod Sahgal, and Guang H. Yue. "From Mental Power to Muscle Power: Gaining Strength by Using the Mind." *Neuropsychologia* 42, no. 7 (February 2004): 944–56. https://lecerveau.mcgill.ca/flash/capsules/articles_pdf/Gaining_strength.pdf.

Taylor, Shelley E., Lien B. Pham, Inna D. Rivkin, and David A. Armor. "Harnessing the Imagination: Mental Simulation, Self-Regulation and Coping." *American Psychologist* 53, no. 4 (April 1998): 429–39. https://www.ncbi.nlm.nih.gov/pubmed/9572006.

Ungerleider, Steven, and Jacqueline Goldin. "Mental Practice among Olympic Athletes." *Perceptual and Motor Skills* 72, no. 3 (1991): 1007–17. https://psycnet.apa.org/record/1992-03652-001.

18. Carefree Karaoke

De Jong, Tania. "10 Reasons to Make Singing Your Happiness Drug." *Huffpost*, December 2014. https://www.huffpost.com/entry/10-reasons-to-make-singing-your-happiness_b_6203630.

Levitin, Daniel J. *This Is Your Brain on Music: The Science of a Human Obsession*. New York: Plume/Penguin, 2013.

Moss, Hilary, Julie Lynch, and Jessica O'Donoghue. "Exploring the Perceived Health Benefits of Singing in a Choir: An International Cross-Sectional Mixed-Methods Study." *Perspectives in Public Health* 138, no. 3 (2018): 160–8. https://www.ncbi.nlm.nih.gov/pubmed/29137545.

Sheppard, Cassandra. "The Neuroscience of Singing." *Uplift*, December 2016. https://upliftconnect.com/neuroscience-of-singing/.

Werber, Cassie. "The Surprising Benefits of Singing at Work." *Quartz*, May 2019. https://qz.com/work/1613520/brits-are-fighting-burnout-by-joining-workplace-choirs/.

19. Mud Pie on Your Face

Edut, Ophira, ed. *Body Outlaws: Rewriting the Rules of Beauty and Body Image*. New York: Seal Press, 2004.

Mrksiy. "Madame Rowley's Toilet Mask." *History 490: Science and Technology in the United States* (blog). September 2016. https://mrksiy .wordpress.com/2016/09/21/madame-rowleys-toilet-mask/.

20. The Power of Twenty

Altucher, James. *Choose Yourself*. Self-published. CreateSpace Independent Publishing Platform, 2013. (*See also Altucher's blog*, The Ultimate Guide for Becoming an Idea Machine *at https://jamesaltucher .com/blog/the-ultimate-guide-for-becoming-an-idea-machine/.*)

Bailey, Chris. *Hyperfocus: How to Be More Productive in a World of Distraction*. New York: Viking, 2018.

Hall, Doug. *Jumpstart Your Brain*. Cincinnati, OH: Clerisy Press, 2007.

Stevenson, Herb. "The Power of Brain Storming: Divergent/Convergent Processes." *Cleveland Consulting Group, Inc.* August, 2017. http://www .clevelandconsultinggroup.com/articles/brain-storming.php.

21. Dances with Bellies

Allred, Terri. *I Belly Dance Because: The Transformative Power of Dance*. Self-published, Xlibris, 2014.

Bräuninger, Iris. "The Efficacy of Dance Movement Therapy Group on Improvement of Quality of Life: A Randomized Controlled Trial." *The Arts in Psychotherapy* 39, no. 4 (2012): 296–303. https://www .sciencedirect.com/science/article/pii/S0197455612000329.

Lewis, Annette C., Sally Davenport, Amelia Hall, and Peter Lovatt. "Mood Changes following Social Dance Sessions in People with Parkinson's Disease." *Journal of Health Psychology* 21, no. 4 (2016): 483–92. https://www.ncbi.nlm.nih.gov/pubmed/24752558.

Lovatt, Peter. "Can Dancing Change the Way We Think?" Filmed November 2011 in London, U.K. TEDxObserver video, 20:33. https:// youtu.be/nDC7Jpf8f4E.

Tucker, Ian. "Peter Lovatt: Dancing Can Change the Way You Think." *The Guardian*, July 2011. https://www.theguardian.com/technology/2011/ jul/31/peter-lovatt-dance-problem-solving.

22. Change Your Clothes, Change Your Life

Hannover, Bettina, and Ulrich Kühnen. "'The Clothing Makes the Self' via Knowledge Activation." *Journal of Applied Social Psychology* 32, no. 12 (2002): 2513-25. https://doi.org/10.1111/j.1559-1816.2002.tb02754.x.

Movinga. "Wasteful World: How Much of Our Belongings Are We Really Using?" Movinga (website). Accessed June 20, 2019. https://www.movinga.de/en/wasteful-world-delusion-reality.

Pine, Karen J. "Happiness: It's Not in the Jeans." Press release summary of survey research from website karenpine.com. http://karenpine.com/wp-content/uploads/2012/03/PR-Happiness-its-not-in-the-jeans.pdf.

———. *Mind What You Wear: The Psychology of Fashion*. Self-published, Amazon Digital Services, 2014. Kindle.

Savasuk, Stasia. "Dressing for Confidence and Joy." Filmed September 2018 in Portsmouth, New Hampshire. TEDxPortsmouth video, 17:35. https://www.youtube.com/watch?v=L5n3VOVYGNg.

Slepian, Michael, Simon N. Ferber, Joshua M. Gold, and Abraham M. Rutchick. "The Cognitive Consequences of Formal Clothing." *Social Psychological and Personality Science* 6, no. 6 (2015): 661-8. http://www.columbia.edu/~ms4992/Publications/2015_Slepian-Ferber-Gold-Rutchick_Clothing-Formality_SPPS.pdf.

Woolf, Virginia. *Orlando*. London: Random House, 2016.

23. A Friendly Q&A

Aron, Arthur, Edward Melinat, Elaine N. Aron, Robert Darrin Valone, and Renee J. Bator. "The Experimental Generation of Interpersonal Closeness: A Procedure and Some Preliminary Findings." *Personality and Social Psychology Bulletin* 23, no. 4 (1997): 363-77. https://journals.sagepub.com/doi/pdf/10.1177/0146167297234003.

Catron, Mandy Len. *How to Fall in Love with Anyone: A Memoir in Essays*. New York: Simon and Schuster, 2017.

———. "To Fall in Love with Anyone, Do This." *New York Times*, January 2015. https://www.nytimes.com/2015/01/11/fashion/modern-love-to-fall-in-love-with-anyone-do-this.html.

McFarlane, Eveyln, and James Saywell. *If: Questions for the Game of Life*. New York: Villard, 1995.

Morris, Margaret E., and Sherry Turkle. *Left to Our Own Devices: Outsmarting Smart Technology to Reclaim Our Relationships, Health, and Focus*. Cambridge, MA: Massachusetts Institute of Technology, 2018.

Stock, Gregory. *The Book of Questions: Revised and Updated*. New York: Workman Publishing, 2013.

Turkle, Sherry. *Alone Together: Why We Expect More from Technology and Less from Each Other*. New York: Basic Books, 2012.

———. *Reclaiming Conversation: The Power of Talk in a Digital Age*. New York: Penguin, 2015.

24. This Playlist Is Me

Lee, Jin-Hyung. "The Effects of Music on Pain: A Meta-analysis." *Journal of Music Therapy* 53, no. 4 (2016): 430–77. https://www.ncbi.nlm.nih.gov/pubmed/27760797.

Levitin, Daniel J. *This Is Your Brain on Music: The Science of a Human Obsession*. New York: Penguin, 2006.

Mannes, Elena. *The Power of Music: Pioneering Discoveries in the New Science of Song*. New York: Bloomsbury, 2013.

Neal, Conan. "'The Power of Music' to Affect the Brain: Interview with Author Elena Mannes." NPR, *Talk of the Nation*, June 2011, 30:17. https://www.npr.org/2011/06/01/136859090/the-power-of-music-to-affect-the-brain.

Picoult, Jodi. *Sing You Home*. New York: Atria Books, 2011.

Prickett, Carol A., and Randall S. Moore. "The Use of Music to Aid Memory of Alzheimer's Patients." *Journal of Music Therapy* 28, no. 2 (1991): 101–10. https://doi.org/10.1093/jmt/28.2.101.

25. Draw on This

De Botton, Alain, and John Armstrong. *Art as Therapy*. London: Phaidon Press, 2016.

Kistler, Mark. *You Can Draw in 30 Days: The Fun, Easy Way to Learn to Draw in One Month or Less*. Philadelphia: Da Capo Press, 2011.

———. *You Can Draw It in Just 30 Minutes: See It and Sketch It in a Half-Hour or Less*. Philadelphia: Da Capo Lifelong Books, 2017.

Urban, Tim, and Andrew Finn. *Wait but Why*. Accessed June 3, 2019. https://waitbutwhy.com.

26. A Friendly Time Capsule

Gibbens, Sarah. "Secret Message Discovered in Statue of Jesus." *National Geographic*, December 2017. https://news.nationalgeographic.com/2017/12/letters-found-butt-jesus-statue-time-capsule-spain-spd/.

Jarvis, William. *Time Capsules: A Cultural History*. Jefferson, NC: McFarland Publishing, 2002.

27. Ages Eight and Up

Barr, Julie. "MIT's LEGO Legacy: Iconic Toy Maker Supports Learning through Play." *MIT Technology Review*. December 2017. https://www.technologyreview.com/s/609588/mits-lego-legacy/.

Johnson, Steven. *Wonderland: How Play Made the Modern World*. New York: Riverhead Books, 2016.

Poon, Linda. "Using Legos as a Legitimate Urban Planning Tool: MIT Wants to Make Transportation Planning More Transparent—and a Bit More Fun." *CityLab*, October 16, 2015. https://www.citylab.com/life/2015/10/legos-as-a-legitimate-urban-planning-tool/410608/.

28. Standing Jokes

Bennett, Mary Payne, and Cecile Lengacher. "Humor and Laughter May Influence Health and Immune Function." *Evidence-Based Complementary and Alternative Medicine* 6, no. 2 (2009): 159–64. https://www.ncbi.nlm.nih.gov/pmc/articles/PMC2686627/.

Miller, Michael, Charles Mangano, Y. Park, Radha Goel, Gary D. Plotnick, and Robert A. Vogel. "Impact of Cinematic Viewing on Endothelial Function." *Heart* 92, no. 2 (2006): 261–2. https://www.ncbi.nlm.nih.gov/pmc/articles/PMC1860773/.

Strean, William B. "Laughter Prescription." *Canadian Family Physician* 55, no. 10 (2009): 965–7. https://www.ncbi.nlm.nih.gov/pmc/articles/PMC2762283/.

Woodward, Jenny. "Jerry Seinfeld: How to Write a Joke." *New York Times Magazine*, video 5:02, December 2012. https://www.nytimes.com/video/magazine/100000001965963/jerry-seinfeld-how-to-write-a-joke-.html.

**And, some of our favorite women comedians
do stand-up for your viewing pleasure:**

Schumer, Amy. *Growing*. Netflix. Released April 2019, filmed December 2018, Chicago Theatre, Chicago Illinois. Runtime 60 minutes.

Sykes, Wanda. *Not Normal*. Netflix. Released May 2019, filmed September 2018, Warner Theatre, Washington D.C. Runtime 60 minutes.

Wong, Ali. *Ali Wong: Baby Cobra*. Netflix. Released May 2016, filmed September 2015, Seattle, Washington. Runtime 60 minutes.

———. *Hard Knock Wife*. Netflix. Released May 2018, filmed September 2017, Toronto's Winter Garden Theatre. Runtime 64 minutes.

29. May I Have a Word?

Boren, Cindy. "Magic Johnson's Stunning Bombshell Was Classic Magic Johnson," *Washington Post*, April 10, 2019. https://www.washingtonpost.com/sports/2019/04/10/magic-johnsons-stunning-bombshell-was-classic-magic-johnson/.

Brysbaert, Marc, Michaël Stevens, Pawel Mandera, and Emmanuel Keuleers. "How Many Words Do We Know? Practical Estimates of Vocabulary Size Dependent on Word Definition, the Degree of Language Input and the Participant's Age." *Frontiers in Psychology* 7 (2016): 1116. https://www.ncbi.nlm.nih.gov/pmc/articles/PMC4965448/.

Ferro, Shaunacy. "The Science behind Why People Hate the Word Moist." *Mental Floss*, June 2015. http://mentalfloss.com/article/64984/science-behind-why-people-hate-word-moist

Konnikova, Maria. "Why Your Name Matters." *New Yorker*, December 19, 2013. https://www.newyorker.com/tech/annals-of-technology/why-your-name-matters.

Merriam-Webster. "We Added New Words to the Dictionary in April 2019: More Than 640 New Words, from 'Bioabsorbable' to 'Bottle Episode.'" *Merriam-Webster*, April 23, 2019. https://www.merriam-webster.com/words-at-play/new-words-in-the-dictionary.

Steelman, Liz. "Do You Know More Words Than the Average American?" *Real Simple*, September 21, 2016. https://www.realsimple.com/work-life/technology/communication-etiquette/how-many-words-english-language-test.

Thibodeau, Paul, Christopher Bromberg, Robby Hernandez, and Zachary Wilson. "An Exploratory Investigation of Word Aversion." *Proceedings of the Annual Meeting of the Cognitive Science Society*, July 2014. Conference paper.

30. Collage Life

Massie, Claudia. "The Women Who Invented Collage—Long before Picasso and Co." *The Spectator*, July 2019. https://www.spectator .co.uk/2019/07/the-women-who-invented-collage-long-before-picasso-and-co/.

Reszies, Heidi. "Scissors, Paper, Glue: Collage and the Making of Poems." *The Volta*, June 2015. http://www.thevolta.org/ewc54-hreszies-p1 .html#note6ref.

Waldman, Diane. *Collage, Assemblage, and the Found Object*. New York: Harry N. Abrams Inc., 1992.

31. A Night at the Improv

Csikszentmihalyi, Mihaly. *Flow: The Psychology of Optimal Experience*. New York: Harper Perennial Modern Classics, 2007.

Kaufman, Sarah L., Jayne Orenstein, Sarah Hashemi, Elizabeth Hart, and Shelly Tan. "Art in an Instant: The Secrets of Improvisation." *Washington Post*, June 2018. https://www.washingtonpost.com/2018/ lifestyle/science-behind-improv-performance/.

32. Close-Knit Friends

Bailey, Chris. "How Learning to Knit Helped My Productivity." *A Life of Productivity Blog*, September 18, 2018. https://alifeofproductivity .com/learning-to-knit-helped-my-productivity/.

———. *Hyperfocus: How to Be More Productive in a World of Distractions*. New York: Random House, 2018.

Barron, Carrie, and Alton Barron. *The Creativity Cure: How to Build Happiness with Your Own Two Hands*. New York: Scribner, 2012.

Brodie, Jane. "The Health Benefits of Knitting." *New York Times Well Blog*, January 25, 2016. https://well.blogs.nytimes.com/2016/01/25/ the-health-benefits-of-knitting/.

Byron, Ellen. "In Mindful Knitting, It's the Journey, Not the Scarf." *Wall Street Journal*, May 21, 2019. https://www.wsj.com/articles/ help-for-stressed-out-workers-mindful-knitting-11558449116.

Geda, Yonas, Hillary M. Topazian, Robert A. Lewis, Rosebud O. Roberts, David S. Knopman, V. Shane Pankratz, Teresa J.H. Christianson, et al. "Engaging in Cognitive Activities, Aging, and Mild Cognitive Impairment: A Population-Based Study." *Journal of Neuropsychiatry and Clinical Neuroscience* 23, no. 2 (2011): 149–54. https://www.ncbi .nlm.nih.gov/pubmed/21677242.

Riley, Jill, Betsan Corkhill, and Morris Clare. "The Benefits of Knitting for Personal and Social Wellbeing in Adulthood: Findings from an International Survey." *The British Journal of Occupational Therapy* 7, no. 2 (February 2013): 50–7. https://doi.org/10.4276/030802 213X13603244419077.

Ritschel, Chelsea. "Knitting Can Reduce Anxiety, Depression, Chronic Pain and Slow Dementia, Research Reveals." *Independent*, March 13, 2018. https://www.independent.co.uk/life-style/knitting-reduces-anxiety-depression-chronic-pain-slows-dementia-research-knit-for-peace-uk-a8254341.html.

Segal, Corinne. "Stitch by Stitch, a Brief History of Knitting and Activism." *PBS.org*, April 23, 2017. https://www.pbs.org/newshour/arts/stitch-stitch-history-knitting-activism.

And one of the many resources online for learning to knit:

KnittingHelp.com. "How to Knit: A Complete Introduction for Beginners Part 1." Duration 19:35. https://knittinghelp.com/video/play/how-to-knit-basics-beginner-tutorial-part-1.

33. And Now for Something *Completely* Different

Bunzeck, Nico, and Emrah Düzel. "Absolute Coding of Stimulus Novelty in the Human Substantia Nigra/VTA." *Neuron* 51, no. 3 (2006): 369–79. https://www.ncbi.nlm.nih.gov/pubmed/16880131.

Wallace, David Foster. "Shipping Out: On the (Nearly Lethal) Comforts of a Luxury Cruise." *Harper's Magazine*, January 1996. https://harpers .org/wp-content/uploads/2008/09/HarpersMagazine-1996-01-0007859.pdf.

34. Move Ya Body

Blackburn, Elizabeth, and Elissa Epel. *The Telomere Effect: A Revolutionary Approach to Living Younger, Healthier, Longer.* New York: Grand Central Publishing, 2018.

Chekroud, Sammi R., Ralitza Gueorguieva, Amanda B. Zheutlin, Martin Paulus, Harlan M. Krumholz, and John H. Krystal. "Association between Physical Exercise and Mental Health in 1.2 Million Individuals in the USA between 2011 and 2015: A Cross-Sectional Study." *Lancet Psychiatry* 5, no. 9 (September 2018): 739–46. https://www.ncbi.nlm.nih.gov/pubmed/30099000.

Crowley, Chris, and Henry S. Lodge. *Younger Next Year: Live Strong, Fit, and Sexy—Until You're 80 and Beyond.* New York: Workman Publishing Company, 2007.

Raichlen, David A., Herman Pontzer, J.A. Harris, Audax Z. Mabulla, Frank W. Marlowe, Jerry Snodgrass, Geeta Eick, Colette Berbesque, Amelia Sancilio, and Brian M. Wood. "Physical Activity Patterns and Biomarkers of Cardiovascular Disease in Hunter-Gatherers." *American Journal of Human Biology* 29, no. 2 (October 2016): e22919. https://www.ncbi.nlm.nih.gov/pubmed/27723159.

Ratey, John. *Spark: The Revolutionary New Science of Exercise and the Brain.* New York: Little, Brown and Company, 2008.

Reynolds, Gretchen. "Born to Move." *New York Times*, November 2016. https://www.nytimes.com/2016/11/23/well/move/born-to-move.html.

35. Local Roots

Bharucha, Zareen P., Netta Weinstein, Dave Watson, and Steffen Boehm. "Participation in Local Food Projects Is Associated with Better Psychological Well-Being: Evidence from the East of England," *Journal of Public Health* (July 2019): fdz057. https://doi.org/10.1093/pubmed/fdz057.

Smith, Alisa, and J.B. MacKinnon. *The 100-Mile Diet: A Year of Local Eating.* Toronto: Vintage Canada, 2007.

USDA. Farmers Markets and Direct-to-Consumer Marketing (website). Accessed June 20, 2019. https://www.ams.usda.gov/sites/default/files/media/NationalCountofFMDirectory17.JPG.

36. Testing the Waters

Mayo Clinic Staff. "Want to Stay Hydrated? Drink before You're Thirsty." Mayo Clinic (website). September 14, 2018. https://www.mayoclinic .org/want-to-stay-hydrated-drink-before-youre-thirsty/art-20390077.

Nichols, Wallace J. *Blue Mind: The Surprising Science That Shows How Being Near, In, On, or Under Water Can Make You Happier, Healthier, More Connected, and Better at What You Do.* New York: Little, Brown and Company, 2014.

United Nations. *The Right to Water: Fact Sheet No. 35.* Accessed June 20, 2019. https://www.ohchr.org/Documents/Publications/ FactSheet35en.pdf.

37. The Dinner of Truth

Anwar, Yasmin. "Is That Stranger Trustworthy? You'll Know in 20 Seconds." *Greater Good Magazine*, November 15, 2011. https:// greatergood.berkeley.edu/article/item/is_that_stranger_trustworthy_ youll_know_in_20_seconds.

Eurich, Tasha. *Insight: The Surprising Truth about How Others See Us, How We See Ourselves and Why the Answers Matter More Than We Think.* New York: Currency, 2018.

38. Biker Chicks

Jag, Julie. "This Is Your Brain on Bikes." *Santa Cruz Sentinel*, April 13, 2019. https://www.santacruzsentinel.com/2019/04/13/this-is-your-brain-on-bikes-sea-otter-classic/.

Macy, Sue. *Wheels of Change: How Women Rode the Bicycle to Freedom (With a Few Flat Tires along the Way).* Washington, D.C.: National Geographic Children's Books, 2017.

Murdoch, Iris. *The Red and the Green.* New York: Penguin, 1967.

Popova, Maria. "A List of Don'ts for Women on Bicycles Circa 1895." *Brainpickings.org*, January 2012. https://www.brainpickings.org/ 2012/01/03/donts-for-women-on-bicycles-1895/.

——. "Wheels of Change: How the Bicycle Empowered Women." *The Atlantic.* March 28, 2011. https://www.theatlantic.com/ technology/archive/2011/03/wheels-of-change-how-the-bicycle-empowered-women/73102/.

39. The Friendly Picnic Society

Williams, Florence. *The Nature Fix: Why Nature Makes Us Happier, Healthier, and More Creative.* New York: W.W. Norton and Company, 2018.

40. The Tea Party Rebellion

Blakemore, Erin. "The Women's Suffrage Movement Started with a Tea Party," *History*, July 10, 2018. https://www.history.com/news/early-womens-rights-suffrage-seneca-falls-elizabeth-cady-stanton.

MacFarlane, Iris, and Alan MacFarlane. *The Empire of Tea: The Remarkable History of the Plant That Took Over the World.* New York: The Overlook Press, 2004.

Pettigrew, Jane. *A Social History of Tea: Tea's Influence on Commerce, Culture & Community.* London: Benjamin Press, 2013.

41. Let's Go Retro!

Langer, Ellen. *Counter Clockwise: Mindful Health and the Power of Possibility.* New York: Ballantine Books, 2009.

McDonald, Tom. "The Young Ones: Can Re-living Your Youth Make You Young Again?" *BBC TV Blog.* September 14, 2010. https://www.bbc.co.uk/blogs/tv/2010/09/the-young-ones.shtml.

42. May I Have a Volunteer?

Killam, Kasley. "A Solution for Loneliness," *Scientific American*, May 21, 2019. https://www.scientificamerican.com/article/a-solution-for-loneliness/.

Lee, Cynthia. "UCLA Marketing Prof Probes What Will Make You Happier: Is It More Time or More Money?" *UCLA Newsroom*, December 2016. http://newsroom.ucla.edu/stories/ucla-prof-finds-out-what-will-make-you-happier.

Lewis, Blair. *Happiness: The Real Medicine and How It Works.* Honesdale, PA: Himalayan Institute Press, 2005.

Luks, Allan. *The Healing Power of Doing Good.* Lincoln, NE: iUniverse.com, 2002.

McGarvey, Amy, Véronique Jochum, John Davies, Joy Dobbs, and
Lisa Hornung. *Time Well Spent: A National Survey on the Volunteer
Experience*, NCVO, January 2019. https://www.ncvo.org.uk/images/
documents/policy_and_research/volunteering/Volunteer-experience_
Full-Report.pdf.

Mogilner, Cassie. "You'll Feel Less Rushed If You Give Time Away."
Harvard Business Review. September 2012. https://hbr.org/2012/09/
youll-feel-less-rushed-if-you-give-time-away.

Ornstein, Robert, and David Sobel. "Psycho-Immunity." *Washington
Post*. May 3, 1987. https://www.washingtonpost.com/archive/
opinions/1987/05/03/psycho-immunity/8455cd33-5e65-4ac9-949a-
9b5210ff0aef/?utm_term=.12b3bc46908b.

Sullivan, G.B., and M.J. Sullivan. "Promoting Wellness in Cardiac
Rehabilitation: Exploring the Role of Altruism." *Journal of
Cardiovascular Nursing* 11, no. 3 (1997): 43–52. https://www.ncbi.nlm
.nih.gov/pubmed/9095453.

UnitedHealthcare/VolunteerMatch. *Do Good Live Well Study: Reviewing the
Benefits of Volunteering*. March 2010. https://cdn.volunteermatch
.org/www/about/UnitedHealthcare_VolunteerMatch_Do_Good_Live_
Well_Study.pdf.

43. Friends Immersion

PBS. *The Science of Healing with Dr. Esther Sternberg*. DVD, 60 minutes.
Resolution Pictures, 2009.

Sternberg, Esther. *The Balance Within: The Science Connecting Health and
Emotions*. New York: W.H. Freeman, 2001.

44. An Act of Faith

Chen, Ying, and Tyler VanderWeele. "Associations of Religious
Upbringing with Subsequent Health and Well-Being from
Adolescence to Young Adulthood: An Outcome-Wide Analysis."
American Journal of Epidemiology 87, no. 11 (2018): 2355–64. https://
doi.org/10.1093/aje/kwy142.

Gyastso, Tenzin (aka the Dalai Lama). "Many Faiths, One Truth." *New
York Times*, May 24, 2010. https://www.nytimes.com/2010/05/25/
opinion/25gyatso.html.

Hartford Institute for Religion Research. "Fast Facts about American Religion." Hartford Institute for Religion Research (website). Accessed June 20, 2019. http://hirr.hartsem.edu/research/fastfacts/fast_facts.html.

Lewis, C.S. "Meditation in a Toolshed." Originally published in *The Coventry Evening Telegraph* (July 17, 1945). http://ktf.cuni.cz/~lin-hb7ak/Meditation-in-a-Toolshed.pdf.

ReligionFacts. "The Big Religion Chart." ReligionFacts (website). Updated November 21, 2016. http://www.religionfacts.com/big-religion-chart.

Solan, Matthew. "Back to School: Learning a New Skill Can Slow Cognitive Aging." *Harvard Health Blog*, April 2016. https://www.health.harvard.edu/blog/learning-new-skill-can-slow-cognitive-aging-201604279502.

VanderWeele, Tyler J. "Religion and Health: A Synthesis." In John Peteet and Michael Balboni, eds., *Spirituality and Religion within the Culture of Medicine: From Evidence to Practice*. New York: Oxford University Press, 2017. http://pik.fas.harvard.edu/files/pik/files/chapter.pdf.

VanderWeele, Tyler J., and John Siniff. "Religion May Be a Miracle Drug: Column." USA *Today*, October 28, 2016. https://www.usatoday.com/story/opinion/2016/10/28/religion-church-attendance-mortality-column/92676964/.

45. Live and Let's Learn

Arnovitz, Kevin. "Pythons and Powerpoints: How the Sixers Cracked the Culture Code." ESPN (website). April 19, 2018. https://www.espn.com/nba/story/_/id/23216496/nba-how-philadelphia-76ers-formed-culture-built-win.

Cassilhas, Ricardo, Sergio Tufik, and Marco Túlio de Mello. "Physical Exercise, Neuroplasticity, Spatial Learning and Memory." *Cellular and Molecular Life Sciences* 73, no. 5 (December 2015): 975–83. https://www.ncbi.nlm.nih.gov/pubmed/26646070.

Delbanco, Andrew. *College: What It Was, Is, and Should Be*. Princeton: Princeton University Press, 2012.

Fiorella, Logan, and Richard E. Mayer. "Role of Expectations and Explanations in Learning by Teaching." *Contemporary Educational Psychology* 39, no. 2 (2014): 75–85. https://doi.org/10.1016/j.cedpsych.2014.01.001.

Gino, Francesca. "Why Curiosity Matters: The Business Case for Curiosity." *Harvard Business Review*, September–October 2018. https://hbr.org/2018/09/curiosity.

Gladwell, Malcolm. "Choice, Happiness and Spaghetti Sauce." Filmed February 2004. TED video, 17:27. https://www.ted.com/talks/malcolm_gladwell_on_spaghetti_sauce?language=en.

Noonan, Susan J. *Managing Your Depression: What You Can Do to Feel Better*. Baltimore: Johns Hopkins University Press, 2013.

Roach, Mary. "10 Things You Didn't Know about Orgasm." Filmed February 2009. TED video, 16:29. https://www.ted.com/talks/mary_roach_10_things_you_didn_t_know_about_orgasm?language=en.

Robson, David. "The Secrets of the 'High-Potential' Personality." BBC *Capital*, May 9, 2018. http://www.bbc.com/capital/story/20180508-the-secrets-of-the-high-potential-personality.

Rowe, John Wallis, and Robert L. Kahn. *Successful Aging*. New York: Dell, 1999. (*This book delves into the results of the MacArthur Foundation study*.)

Thomas, Ed. "Kenyan Grandmother at School with Her Great-Great-Grandchildren." BBC *News*, January 23, 2015. https://www.bbc.com/news/world-africa-30935874.

Waldinger, Robert. "What Makes a Good life? Lessons from the Longest Study on Happiness." Filmed November 2015. TEDxBeaconStreet video, 12:47. https://www.ted.com/talks/robert_waldinger_what_makes_a_good_life_lessons_from_the_longest_study_on_happiness?language=en.

Zhang, Chen, Christopher G. Myers, and David M. Mayer. "To Cope with Stress, Try Learning Something New." *Harvard Business Review*, September 4, 2018. https://hbr.org/2018/09/to-cope-with-stress-try-learning-something-new.

Zipkin, Nina. "Watch Oprah Winfrey's Empowering 2018 USC Commencement Speech" (Transcript). *Entrepreneur*. May 2018. https://www.entrepreneur.com/article/313386.

46. A Grave Matter

Berendt, John. *Midnight in the Garden of Good and Evil*. New York: Random House, 1994.

Crowther, Linnea. "Why Cemeteries Are Important." Legacy.com (website). 2015. http://www.legacy.com/news/culture-and-trends/article/why-cemeteries-are-important.

Gailliot, Matthew, Tyler Stillman, Brandon Schmeichel, Jon K. Maner, and E. Ashby Plant. "Mortality Salience Increases Adherence to Salient Norms and Values." *Personal and Social Psychology Bulletin* 34, no. 7 (May 9, 2008): 993-1003. https://www.ncbi.nlm.nih.gov/pubmed/18550864.

Weiss, John P. "Three Reasons You Need to Visit a Graveyard." The Good Men Project (website). January 2, 2015. https://goodmenproject.com/featured-content/three-reasons-you-need-to-visit-a-graveyard-hesaid/.

47. Put Slumber Back in the Party

Al Khatib, Haya, Scott V. Harding, Julia Darzi, and Gerda K. Pot. "The Effects of Partial Sleep Deprivation on Energy Balance: A Systematic Review and Meta-analysis." *European Journal of Clinical Nutrition* 71, no. 2 (2016): 614-24. https://www.ncbi.nlm.nih.gov/pubmed/27804960.

Cohen, Sheldon, William J. Doyle, Cuneyt M. Alper, Denise Janicki-Deverts, and Ronald B. Turner. "Sleep Habits and Susceptibility to the Common Cold." *Archives of Internal Medicine, American Medical Association* 169, no. 1 (2009): 62-7. https://www.ncbi.nlm.nih.gov/pmc/articles/PMC2629403/.

Holding, Benjamin C., Tina Sundelin, Patrick Cairns, David I. Perrett, and John Axelsson. "The Effect of Sleep Deprivation on Objective and Subjective Measures of Facial Appearance." *Journal of Sleep Research* (April 2019): e12860. https://doi.org/10.1111/jsr.12860.

Huffington, Arianna. *The Sleep Revolution*. New York: Harmony, 2017.

Liu, Yong, Anne G. Wheaton, Daniel P. Chapman, Timothy J. Cunningham, Hua Lu, and Janet B. Croft. "Prevalence of Healthy Sleep Duration among Adults—United States, 2014." *Morbidity Mortality Weekly Report* 65, no. 6 (2016): 137-41. https://www.cdc.gov/mmwr/volumes/65/wr/mm6506a1.htm.

Walker, Matthew. "Sleep Is Your Superpower." Filmed April 2019, Vancouver, British Columbia. TEDTalk video, 19:19. https://www.youtube.com/watch?v=5MuIMqhT8DM.

Walker, Matthew. *Why We Sleep: Unlocking the Power of Sleep and Dreams*. New York: Scribner, 2017.

About the Authors

LYNNE EVERATT is a recovering MBA, a LinkedIn Top Voice in management and culture, and an ardent advocate for wellness through physical fitness. As part of her MBA recovery, she wrote *The 5-Minute Recharge: 31 Proven Strategies to Refresh, Reset and Become the Boss of Your Day*, aimed at improving workplace mental health, and *Emails from the Edge*, which was nominated for the Stephen Leacock Medal for Humour. Prior to pursuing her dream of becoming a writer, Lynne worked with numbers at a multinational pharmaceutical company where she met co-authors Deb Mangolt and Julie Smethurst, who share her love of physical activity, earthy food, and personal growth through friendship.

DEB MANGOLT'S positive attitude and bubbly personality are ideally suited to helping others get the most out of life, and as a former finance director at a Fortune 500 company, she reinvented herself to better express her strengths. An event planner, life coach, dance fitness instructor, and a cherished friend to many, Deb inspires others to become the best versions of who they are. As an avid golfer, Deb is grateful for having "the best of both worlds," living in Florida in the winter and on Muskoka Bay, Ontario, in the summer, with her husband, Randy.

JULIE SMETHURST loves her life devoted to family and her passions, and strives to make a difference through the work she does. But this hasn't always been the case. After obtaining her CPA, Julie spent two decades climbing the corporate ladder only to find her life was out of balance. With a deep longing to live a life true to herself, she looked to friends Lynne and Deb to help her transform. Julie chucked the full-time job, adapted her ways of working, created dedicated family time, and pursued her desires to learn to fly and play tennis and golf. She even indulged her love of all things French by studying the language. She has a passion for healthy food and enjoys taking long walks and bike rides with her husband.

Together, LYNNE, DEB, AND JULIE are on a mission to encourage women to discover new ways to raise each other up through friendship, just as they have discovered the best in themselves through each other.

actsoffriendship.com